DECISION-MAKING IN NURSING

Thoughtful Approaches for Leadership

SECOND EDITION

Edited by

Sandra B. Lewenson, EdD, RN, FAAN
Professor of Nursing
College of Health Professions
Lienhard School of Nursing
Pace University
Pleasantville, New York

Marie Truglio-Londrigan, PhD, RN
Professor of Nursing
College of Health Professions
Lienhard School of Nursing
Pace University
Pleasantville, New York

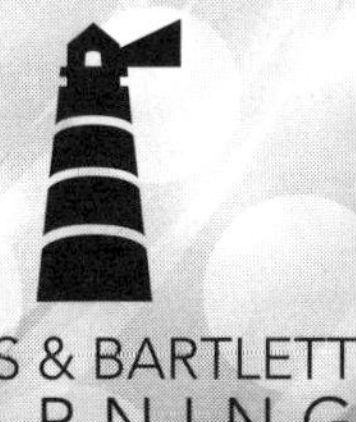

JONES & BARTLETT
LEARNING

World Headquarters
Jones & Bartlett Learning
5 Wall Street
Burlington, MA 01803
978-443-5000
info@jblearning.com
www.jblearning.com

Jones & Bartlett Learning books and products are available through most bookstores and online booksellers. To contact Jones & Bartlett Learning directly, call 800-832-0034, fax 978-443-8000, or visit our website, www.jblearning.com.

Substantial discounts on bulk quantities of Jones & Bartlett Learning publications are available to corporations, professional associations, and other qualified organizations. For details and specific discount information, contact the special sales department at Jones & Bartlett Learning via the above contact information or send an email to specialsales@jblearning.com.

Production Credits
Executive Publisher: William Brottmiller
Senior Editor: Amanda Martin
Associate Acquisitions Editor: Teresa Reilly
Associate Managing Editor: Sara Bempkins
Production Editor: Keith Henry
Marketing Communications Manager: Katie Hennessy
VP, Manufacturing and Inventory Control: Therese Connell
Composition: Laserwords Private Limited, Chennai, India
Cover Design: Kristin E. Parker
Cover Image: © antishock/ShutterStock, Inc.
Printing and Binding: Edwards Brothers Malloy
Cover Printing: Edwards Brothers Malloy

Library of Congress Cataloging-in-Publication Data
Decision-making in nursing : thoughtful approaches for leadership /
[edited by] Sandra B. Lewenson and Marie Truglio-Londrigan.—Second edition.
p. ; cm.
Includes bibliographical references and index.
ISBN 978-1-284-02617-7 (pbk.)
I. Lewenson, Sandra, editor of compilation. II. Truglio-Londrigan,
Marie, editor of compilation.
[DNLM: 1. Decision Making. 2. Nursing Care–methods. 3. Leadership.
WY 100.1]
RT42
610.73—dc23

2013049711

6048

Printed in the United States of America
18 17 16 15 14   10 9 8 7 6 5 4 3 2 1

Contents

Foreword

Angela Barron McBride, PhD, RN, FAAN
Distinguished Professor and
University Dean Emerita
Indiana University School of Nursing

Lewenson and Truglio-Londrigan's first edition of *Decision-Making in Nursing: Thoughtful Approaches to Practice* received a 2008 *American Journal of Nursing* Book of the Year Award. The second edition, retitled *Decision-Making in Nursing: Thoughtful Approaches for Leadership* to reflect the fact that all nurses must see themselves as leaders prepared to make decisions, builds on the originality of the first publication, but expands our notion of decision-making to being an everyday process for selecting the best alternatives from available information. Their preface to the current version begins by reminding us that not all nurses see themselves as leaders, but they all have to move in that direction if they are to deliver—both individually and collectively—the transformational leadership expected of them in the twenty-first century.

This new volume is just what a second edition should be. The first edition came into existence because the editors taught a graduate course entitled "Advanced Decision-Making in Primary Health Care," and no text on that topic existed, despite the fundamental importance of the subject. What they proceeded to piece together was a multidimensional view of decision-making that was particularly good at providing case studies of how each way of knowing enriched the nurse's possibility of finding the best solution. Freed now from the constraints of assembling the basics, this new edition has all of the benefits of the earlier version, but the focus isn't just on the primacy of decision-making to the success of provider–patient relationships, but also decision-making's role in affecting the system change required of all nurses by a host of external factors—constrained resources, the graying of the population, the Affordable Care Act, values-based purchasing, socioeconomic inequities, and so forth. Accordingly, each chapter has been revised to emphasize that decision-making is important to all nurses because it provides a process for selecting the best way to meet the unprecedented challenges of today's clinical environments in which each professional is expected to improve quality and access while bending the cost curve downward.

This edition begins, appropriately and classically, with a chapter on knowing yourself, but then devotes chapters to all of the other ways of knowing that nurses need in order to be effective—a historical perspective, an appreciation of ethical and legal issues, cultural sensitivity, family viewpoints, existing policies, evidence to date, use of technology, and so forth. This version of the book not only creatively explores how decisions are increasingly being made by teams, but also confronts how current economic realities and an assortment of technological advances also influence decisions. The result is a book that prepares nurses not to follow orders, but to take the lead in working appropriately with others to improve the well-being of individuals, families, and communities.

For the nursing profession, the twentieth century was a period of intense infrastructure development (establish graduate programs, research training, standards, etc.), and the emphasis was on the problem-solving or decision-making components of the nursing process because nurses sought to prove that they are competent professionals. Whether nurses are full professionals is no longer in doubt; now the issue is whether they can assume the responsibilities being demanded of them. In the twenty-first century, nurses are expected to exert transformational leadership, with its emphasis on greater decision-making and innovation (IOM, 2004).

Nurses once were prepared to support the primary caregiver; now they are expected to be the primary caregiver capable of managing population-based care. Nurses once only aspired to positions that had the word "nurse" in their titles (e.g., chief nurse officer, school of nursing dean); now they are groomed to exert interprofessional leadership. For example, Marilyn Tavenner heads the Administration for the Centers for Medicare and Medicaid Services (CMS) and Mary Wakefield directs the Health Resources and Services Administration (HRSA).

This second edition is a major stepping stone along the way to preparing new generations for the many decisions they will have to make in the practice of tomorrow.

References

Institute of Medicine (IOM). (2004). *Keeping patients safe: Transforming the work environment of nurses*. Washington, DC: National Academies Press.

Preface

Editors
Sandra B. Lewenson, EdD, RN, FAAN
Marie Truglio-Londrigan, PhD, RN

Strong leadership is critical if the vision of a transformed health care system is to be realized. Yet not all nurses begin their career with thoughts of becoming a leader. The nursing profession must produce leaders throughout the health care system, from the bedside to the boardroom, who can serve as full partners with other health professionals and be accountable for their own contributions to delivering high-quality care while working collaboratively with leaders from other health professions.

—Institute of Medicine, 2011, p. 22

The Institute of Medicine's (IOM) 2011 report, *The Future of Nursing: Leading Change, Advancing Health*, considers nursing a major participant in the decisions that will be made in our healthcare system in the years ahead. The American Association of Colleges of Nursing (2008, 2011) published a revised Baccalaureate Essentials and a Master's Essentials that also speak to nurses being leaders in the changing healthcare setting. All three documents ask that nurses at their respective levels be able to work on interprofessional care teams, translate evidence into practice, and participate in quality and safety initiatives. This requires nurses to be leaders and decision makers. Making decisions in the twenty-first century requires reflective thought, interdisciplinary focus, global perspectives, use of technology, leadership skills, and comfort with ambiguity. Nurses face challenges every day when caring for people. A choice for one person may not be appropriate for another. Factors such as diverse populations, changing healthcare systems, limited resources, and a challenging environment provide some of the reasons why we must look at the different ways we make decisions. Nurses need to critically think through their decisions, be willing to be flexible, and know what they know and what they do not know, as well as be aware of many ways to approach a decision. Nurses need to be reflective of who they are in the context of their patients, families, communities, and populations.

This second edition, newly titled *Decision-Making in Nursing: Thoughtful Approaches for Leadership*, explores the contributions of a variety of decision-making approaches that add to the ways of knowing and the evidence that enable nursing professionals to be reflective, critical, flexible, and comfortable with the many decisions they make on a daily basis. The editors of this book believe that all nurses act as leaders in practice, administration, education, or research and therefore we have renamed this decision-making text to include "leadership" in the title to reflect this belief. This book offers a variety of thoughtful approaches that the practitioner can integrate into his or her practice. The book looks at the various ways in which we make decisions and shows that although the various approaches may be presented independently, they are interdependently connected. Carper (1992) recognized that the various "patterns of knowing" are "not mutually exclusive" and described them as "interrelated and interdependent" (p. 77). We view the various approaches in a similar manner. Although each chapter focuses on a specific approach used in decision-making, it does so for the purpose of allowing the nurse as leader to understand and apply the concepts of this approach in their decisions.

The significance of this book lies in its reflective, multidimensional approach to decision-making. We see the healthcare arena and the care provided as extremely complex and a dynamic process that one can imagine as a "holographic" view of the experience at any given point in time. Depending on the angle you are looking at, the holographic image changes. Nurses looking at a individual, family, community, and population may need to choose a different decision-making approach based on the multidimensional image that is presented at any given moment. Nurses, therefore, must be aware of the many ways in which decisions can be made and implemented in the care of individuals, families, communities, and populations. Nurses require the ability to be fluid in their thinking, which enables them to see and be willing to look at the issues in front of them from different vantage points simultaneously. This means using multiple approaches throughout the decision-making process.

Nurses who practice with a one-dimensional approach to care frequently find their outcomes limited and inconsistent with the philosophical beliefs of nursing. For example, nurses in a county department of health identified that the morbidity and mortality rates for prostate cancer in black males were alarmingly high. These nurses, along with other public health officials, dutifully developed and implemented a public health initiative for the prevention of prostate cancer including early identification and treatment for black men. Their decision to implement this program was based solely on statistical evidence and lacked depth or breadth that would have considered culture, race, ethnicity, family, history, economics, legal and ethical issues, and a myriad of other contextual factors that may have influenced the success of this program. The program did not acknowledge these other factors and therefore failed to meet the desired healthcare outcomes. These nurses lacked a holistic view that nursing claims to hold. They functioned more like Benner's (1984) novice-level nurses and less like experts who typically use a more holistic view. Nevertheless, all nurses need to consider the various approaches that interrelate and are interdependent in their decision-making process. An awareness of the multiple approaches of decision-making would have allowed the public health nurses to expand their decision-making from just the one-model statistical approach to more of a holistic approach. By using an expanded view, they would have taken into account these various factors, reached out, and partnered with this targeted population and other organizations in the community who worked with them. This broader partnership would have allowed the planners to see the intervention strategy in a different way and thus understand the need to expand their worldview when making decisions.

If we look at the use of restraints with the elderly, decisions were made based on what was thought to ensure the safety of the patient; however, decisions were not based on evidence such as history, patient preferences, or ethical concerns. Brush and Capezuti (2001) looked at the era when hospitals first introduced side rails as an intervention strategy to prevent falls. Through their historical research, they found that side rails were first used in the 1930s to prevent falls and possible lawsuits. Nurses did not have evidence nor seek evidence that supported the safety aspect of using siderails. The physical, psychological, ethical, and economic questions surrounding the use of restraints had not been addressed during this early period of time. However, today, the driving force for healthcare decisions is evidence-based. This evidence includes not only empirical data, but also the evidence provided by the historical antecedents.

Leaders make decisions every day; nurses make decisions every day. Nurses lead and accept leadership roles in the clinical settings, in the classroom, in the boardroom, and in research projects (IOM, 2011, p. 221). As a result, it is expected that all nurses lead with patients, with staff, within inter- or intraprofessional teams, in a primary healthcare setting, or in an academic setting. Yet, it is not easy for some nurses to accept the idea that they are a leader, perhaps due to the educational pathway, the image they hold of nursing and themselves, or their own professional maturity. To be a leader and to make the decisions leaders need to make, you are putting yourself out there, where criticism and the risk of failure loom. The chapters in this book set the stage and facilitate a conversation for nurses at any point of care. Nurses have a wide range of skill sets needed by leaders. The ability to be facile in decision-making allows nurses to take ownership of the decisions that need to be made in the care of individuals, families, communities, and populations, as well as decisions on interdisciplinary care teams, within the profession, and in the healthcare environment. Therefore, this book provides nurses and students of nursing the opportunity to see themselves as leaders and feel comfortable making decisions as leaders.

Organization of the Book

The authors felt that nurses needed *Decision-Making in Nursing: Thoughtful Approaches for Leadership* to provide the tools to look at their decision-making as a multidimensional, reflective experience. The book examines how self-reflection, history, legal and ethical issues, spirituality, culture, family, the media, groups, evidence-based practice, economics, technology, and health policy affect the way we make decisions. It offers ways of knowing that nurses can use to critically think through a decision and be the leader that is expected of all nurses.

Although other approaches to decision-making exist, we selected these as important to consider throughout the decision-making process. And although nurses may not use each approach for every decision they make, just being aware of the possibilities allows for the complexity, fluidity, and flexibility in thinking that nurses need.

Each chapter will include at least one case study using a nursing scenario that will illustrate the use of a particular approach in an actual practice setting. We use nursing scenarios as exemplars for several reasons. Nurses represent most of the healthcare professionals in the

United States; there are over 3 million nurses reported in the country. Nurses touch the lives of people in every situation—from birth to death, in health and illness. People turn to nurses to ask questions to make better healthcare decisions. Nurses deal in human responses. Decisions are a human response to a particular situation. Our own backgrounds and the backgrounds of our contributors as nurses and nursing educators provide a rich tapestry from which we can draw. We use this multidimensional reflective approach to better understand the process of decision-making in the healthcare setting. To allow for diversity of ideas, we asked each of the contributors to write from their own experiences as leaders and decision makers and develop their own case studies (as many as they liked). Each of the contributing authors updated their chapters and we added a totally new chapter on economics and decision-making as well as a new chapter on how technology influences decision-making. We also revised our chapter on group decision-making to reflect a shared decision-making approach. The editors believe these additions and revisions in chapters and title of the book offer nurses ways in which to view their decisions in light of their ever-expanding leadership roles in practice.

Chapter 1, "Know Yourself: Reflective Decision-Making," explains the use of self-reflection in the decision-making process. Authors Marie Truglio-Londrigan and Sandra B. Lewenson use themselves as a "case study" in which they present a reflection of who they are and how this may have affected the decisions they have made. The self-reflection that the authors undergo also demonstrates the way they filter the logic and critical thinking that they use when making decisions. Like Durgahee (1996) observes, "knowledge lies within the practical situations" (p. 426). Self-reflection asks that we look at ourselves and transform our everyday life experiences into knowledge that we apply in decision-making. What the authors present is that knowledge lies embedded within everyday life experiences.

Chapter 2, titled "Looking Back: History and Decision-Making in Health Care," discusses how history informs decisions. Author Sandra B. Lewenson looks at the history of decision-making in nursing and examines how nurses have made decisions in the past. It also looks at how the history of the profession itself affects decision-making in the clinical and educational arena. The role of women, modernization of hospitals, and the changing roles of healthcare providers have influenced the kinds of decisions that have been made and continue to be made. Examples of historical studies are used throughout the chapter to explain how important history is to decision-making. The case study used depicts a community assessment looking at historical data from 1893 and how nurses like Lillian Wald made important healthcare decisions on the Lower East Side of New York.

Chapter 3, "Right or Wrong: Policy, Legal and Ethical Issues, and Decision-Making," discusses the legal and ethical issues that inform the healthcare decision-making process. Nurse-attorney Elizabeth Furlong presents an updated case study showing what could have happened if a proposed law in Nebraska passed and the bearing it could have had on nurses' decisions regarding the care of a dying patient. The law would have created tension among the nurses' professional code of ethics, the law, and their own beliefs about care. The contributor provides a discussion about the ethics of caring and how it pertains to the nurses' decision-making process. In addition, this chapter looks at the factors that influence the healthcare professional as they make the determination to alter healthcare policy.

In Chapter 4, "More than Prayer: Spirituality and Decision-Making," noted historian Joy Buck examines spirituality and the affect it has on nurses' ability to make decisions and help patients do the same. The chapter takes into account the patients' spiritual needs, the historical relevance of spirituality and nursing care, and the nurses' ability to understand their own spirituality and that of the patient, family, and community. Buck addresses values, moral distress, religious beliefs, and what is meant by spirituality and decision-making in nursing. Compelling case studies throughout the chapter illustrate the need for nurses to be aware of how the patient's spirituality, as well as their own, influence the decision-making process.

Culture plays an important role in how people respond to issues surrounding sickness and health. Chapter 5, "Culture and Decision-Making," examines the impact culture has on a nurse's decision-making ability. In this chapter, nurse educator Caroline Camuñas examines how the culture of the provider as well as the consumer affect decision-making. Camuñas presents a cogent discussion about organizational culture, various ways of knowing, and the importance of dialogue to understanding culture. The chapter also looks at how the culture of each person in the decision-making process affects the way the decision is made, the actual final decision, and how they, the patient, and the healthcare provider relate to each other. This chapter forces nurses to reflect on who they are, and in so doing, be mindful of their conduct, the decisions they make, and how they relate to their patients, families, and communities.

Family plays a large role in the life of an individual and thus on the decisions surrounding health care. Chapter 6, "Family and Decision-Making," presents case studies that exemplify different families and the need for nurses to be mindful of the needs of each when working with families. Nurse educator Susan Salmond looks at how family members influence a healthcare decision and the need for healthcare providers to be aware of how their own family background and experiences interface with those of their patients.

Chapter 7, "Media and Decision-Making," explores the nature of media and decision-making. Founder of the Truth About Nursing, Sandy Summers, and coauthor Harry Jacobs Summers provide insights about media and techniques media may use that influence healthcare decision-making among professionals and the population at large. Examples are provided of how the media, including television, books, movies, the Internet, and public health campaigns, influences the decisions made about health care. Nursing images in the media such as the "naughty nurse," "battle-ax," and "angel" affect the way nursing decisions are viewed by various populations, including other health professionals, the people nurses serve, and nurses themselves. Nursism, or the bias toward the caring role (Lewenson, 1993), may block an acceptance of nurses as decision makers. Summers and Summers demonstrate how the media can influence both the consumer of health care and the healthcare provider in the process of reflective decision-making. They also provide useful steps that can be taken by nurses to positively influence the messages transmitted by the media.

Chapter 8, "Working Together: Shared Decision-Making," explores the process of shared decision-making in groups, specifically teams and coalitions. The authors of this chapter speak about groups of individuals comprising a team and groups of organizations who partner to form coalitions. Throughout the chapter, the idea of shared decision-making informs the way in which teams and coalitions work within their respective groups. The discussion about using shared decision-making offers a valuable thoughtful approach for nursing leadership. Authors Marie Truglio-Londrigan and Cheryl Barnes enhance the chapter by presenting interesting case studies that illustrate shared decision-making in teams and coalitions.

Nurses make decisions using evidence. This is not a new concept. Nurses have sought evidence through research since the days of Florence Nightingale. Nightingale's use of data to support her work during the Crimean War and Lillian Wald's use of data to support the work of the Henry Street Settlement laid the groundwork for nurses to use evidence to support their work. In Chapter 9, "Evidence-Based Decision-Making," authors Jason Slyer, Catherine Concert, and Joanne Singleton examine the various dimensions of evidence that nurses must gather to make informed decisions for best practice. This chapter includes discussion of systematic reviews, history, patient preferences, and other sources of evidence as nurses engage in decision-making.

Many decisions regarding health care are influenced by economic reality. Nurses need to know and understand how economics drives healthcare decisions. The trick is how nurses use economic data to inform their decisions without compromising the other dimensions of the multidimensional reflective decision-making approaches. In Chapter 10, "Healthcare Costs Matter: Economics and Decision-Making," editor of *Nursing Economic$* and nurse educator, Donna Nickitas addresses the challenges of the Patient Protection and Affordable Care Act as well as what nurses need to know in order to participate in financially driven decisions. Healthcare providers need to understand the concepts behind economic decision-making and the ultimate outcome pertaining to care rendered to individuals, families, communities, and populations.

In Chapter 11, "Getting Involved: Public Policy and Influencing the Outcomes," health policy consultant Judith K. Leavitt and nurse educator and midwife Andréa Sonenberg look at how legislators make decisions, very often influenced by special interest groups and lobbyists. Nurses play an important role by providing lawmakers with knowledge and evidence necessary to make informed decisions with regard to health policy that ultimately has a direct effect on populations. Nurses especially can offer evidence that drives needed policy changes. Focused analyses of issues, community coalitions, and partnerships are all a part of this process necessary to educate and influence policy makers, which is integral to healthcare policy decision-making.

The final approach presented in this text is a new chapter titled "Use of Technology for Decision-Making." Technology plays a major role in how decisions are made now and will be made in the future. Whether through the use of data mining, telehealth, or electronic health records and electronic medical records, nurses at all points of care must be knowledgeable about technology. Even the use of a virtual dog in a research proposal shows the innovative ways in which technology can be used to reduce isolation. This chapter provides a variety of perspectives shared by a group of authors including Christine Malmgreen, Karen Koziol, Angela Northrop, Veronica Elizabeth Francois, Lorraine Von Eeden, Sharon Stahl Wexler, and Lin Drury. The ideas of these authors were linked together based on the editors' conception for this chapter and the wide applications of technology.

Campbell (2004) compiled a definition of *critical thinking* from the literature as "open-minded reasoning; use of intellectual standards of reasoning including, clarity, depth and breadth of understanding and relevance of information to a situation, and questioning of assumptions and biases" (p. 195). The approaches presented in *Decision-Making in Nursing: Thoughtful Approaches for Leadership* offer nurses the tools to entertain the open-minded reasoning that critical thinking requires. The different thoughtful approaches merge as a holographic image and create a multidimensional reflective model. Imagine a holographic image as a visual of what we see as essential to use in decision-making. We also recognize that we cannot include all the infinite number of approaches that one may use in making decisions, but we have selected some that we think are important. Essential to this book is the idea that there is no one best method to use to make a decision. Using any one approach is too linear, too singular, too rigid, and too incomplete to aid nurses in the care of their patients, families, communities, and populations in this increasingly complex world in which we live.

This second edition offers a wider array of ideas both from contributors and from what the authors learned from the first edition. They had used the first edition in a decision-making course where students expressed appreciation for the usability and applicability of the text. As the years progressed and the essential documents for both baccalaureate and master's education changed, the authors embraced this change and drew on the ideas of leadership, teamwork, and inter- and intraprofessional relationships. They expanded and updated the chapters and included one on technology. Yet they still believe that this second edition, like the first, leaves us with more questions than answers on how to make decisions.

References

American Association of Colleges of Nursing (AACN). (2008). *Essentials of baccalaureate nursing education for professional practice*. Washington, DC: AACN.

American Association of Colleges of Nursing (AACN). (2011). *Essentials of master's nursing education for professional practice*. Washington, DC: AACN.

Benner, P. (1984). *From novice to expert: Excellence and power in clinical nursing practice*. Menlo Park, CA: Addison-Wesley.

Brush, B. L., & Capezuti, E. (2001). Historical analysis of siderail use in American hospitals. *Journal of Nursing Scholarship*, 23(4), 381–385.

Campbell, E. T. (2004). Meeting practice challenges via a clinical decision-making course. *Nurse Educator*, 29(5), 195–198.

Carper, B. A. (1992). Philosophical inquiry in nursing: An application. In J. E. Kikuchi & H. Simmons (Eds.), *Philosophical inquiry in nursing* (pp. 71–80). London: Sage Publications.

Durgahee, T. (1996). Promoting reflection in post-graduate nursing: A theoretical model. *Nurse Education Today*, 16, 419–426.

Institute of Medicine (IOM). (2011). *The future of nursing: Leading change, advancing health*. Washington, DC: National Academies Press.

Lewenson, S. B. (1993). *Taking charge: Nursing suffrage, and feminism*, 1873–1920. New York: Garland Press.

About the Authors

Sandra B. Lewenson, EdD, RN, FAAN, is a Professor of Nursing at the College of Health Professions, Lienhard School of Nursing, Pace University. Her research interests include the history of nursing's political activity during the early part of the twentieth century, the establishment of the American Red Cross Rural Public Health Nursing Service, the changing definitions of public health nursing throughout the twentieth and twenty-first centuries, and the change in nursing education from an apprenticeship model to a baccalaureate and higher degree. She has received several awards in nursing including the Outstanding Scholarship and Research Award from Teachers College, Columbia University; Hall of Fame of the Alumni Association of Hunter College; the American Association for the History of Nursing Lavinia Dock Award for Historical Scholarship and Research in Nursing; the *American Journal of Nursing* Book of the Year Award; Sigma Theta Tau's Media Nursing Print Award; and most recently the American Association for the History of Nursing Mary M. Roberts Award. She is a fellow in the American Academy of Nursing and a member of Sigma Theta Tau International Honor Society.

Marie Truglio-Londrigan, PhD, RN, holds a baccalaureate degree from Herbert H. Lehman College, an MSN in primary health care nursing of the aged from Seton Hall University, and a PhD in nursing from Adelphi University. Dr. Truglio-Londrigan has been a nurse since 1976 and has primarily practiced in public health, community, and long-term care. Most recently she has held a faculty practice at Aging in America, the parent company for Morningside House in the Bronx; prior to that she served as a consultant for population-based practice at the Bergen County Department of Health Services in New Jersey. Her practice has focused primarily on the area of public and community, with a specialization in the care of older adults. Presently, Dr. Truglio-Londrigan is a Professor at the College of Health Professions, Lienhard School of Nursing. She is a Fellow of the New York Academy of Medicine and has participated in several evidence-based practice initiatives with Doctor of Nursing Practice (DNP) students. Her own research interests include shared decision-making, health promotion, and disease prevention with an emphasis on patient-centered care.

Acknowledgments

I want to acknowledge the love and support of my family, who helped me think through the writing of this book and offered their opinions freely. Thank you to Richard, my husband, for his unfailing love and support; to my daughters Jenni and Nicky and both their terrific husbands, Chris and Jeff, who encouraged and supported me throughout all the decision-making that needed to be done both at home and in this book; to our three wonderful granddaughters, Georgia, Sarah, and Pearl, who are learning to make decisions every day; and to my brother's family—Billy, Cindy, Heather, Ross, and Barbie—and to my sister Michelle for all being there. I want to offer a special thank you to my colleague and friend, Marie Truglio-Londrigan, for her persistence and belief in this project. And finally, I want to acknowledge the wonderful students who recognize the relevance of decision-making in their leadership role as a nurse.

Sandra B. Lewenson

Identifying that there was a need for this book was easy. The decision to actually engage in the writing process was a difficult one. Once the decision was made, there was a tremendous sense of responsibility to do the job and to do it well. There are many people in my life who have helped me in this process. They have also supported me on a daily basis just by their presence. The first is my husband Michael. Over 45 years ago, he asked me if I wanted to ride our bicycles together. I made a decision that summer day to go with him. This was the best decision of my life. His unwavering support has helped me ever since. Not a day goes by that I do not ask him what he thinks about certain issues, and his guidance is accepted and greatly appreciated. My two children, Paul and Leah, have taught me something in their own way. Those lessons sometimes were hard to take, but I have no doubt they were lessons that I needed to learn. Since the initial writing of this book my two children have married and I now have four children. Jacklyn and Christopher have been added to the familial mix along with their pets, Loki, Orsa, and Ozzie. My hope is that my children will be happy and that as their lives unfold they learn to share in decisions as their father and mother have. To those who have gone before me, I thank you for providing me with memories and a solid foundation that has helped me in my attempt at shaping a meaningful life.

Marie Truglio-Londrigan

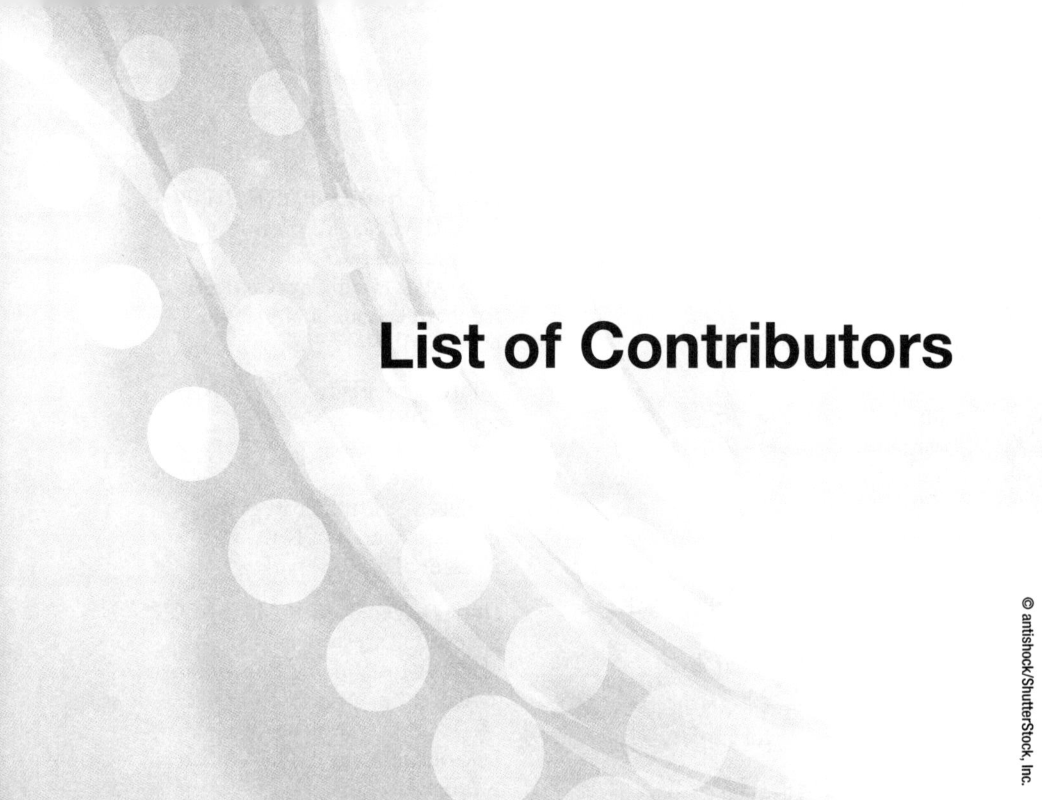

List of Contributors

Cheryl Barnes, DNP, FNP, RN
Nurse Practitioner
Memorial Sloan Kettering Cancer Center
New York, New York

Joy Buck, PhD, RN
Associate Professor
West Virginia University School of Nursing, Eastern Division
Martinsburg, West Virginia

Caroline Camuñas, EdD, RN
Adjunct Associate Professor
Health and Behavior Studies
Nursing Education
Teachers College, Columbia University
New York, New York
Research Coordinator
James J. Peters VA Medical Center
Bronx, New York

Connie M. Concert, DNP, RN, FNP-BC, CGRN
Pace University
College of Health Professions
Lienhard School of Nursing
Senior Nurse Practitioner
Beth Israel Medical Center
New York, New York

Lin Drury, PhD, RN
Associate Professor of Nursing
Pace University
College of Health Professions
Lienhard School of Nursing
New York, New York

Veronica E. Francois, DNP, RN, FNP-BC
Montefiore Medical Center
Department of Radiology/Division of Nuclear Medicine
Bronx, New York

Elizabeth Furlong, RN, PhD, JD
Associate Professor, School of Nursing
Faculty Associate, Center for Health Policy and Ethics
Creighton University
Omaha, Nebraska

Karen Koziol, RNC, MS
Clinical Coordinator
Dominican College
Orangeburg, New York
Information Coordinator
Mercy College
Dobbs Ferry, New York

Judith K. Leavitt, RN, MEd, FAAN
Health Policy Consultant
Barnardsville, North Carolina

Christine Malmgreen, RN-BC, MA, MSN
Associate Director for Professional Practice
Hudson Valley Hospital Center
Cortland Manor, New York

Donna M. Costello Nickitas, PhD, RN, NEA-BC, CNE, FNAP, FAAN
Professor and Executive Officer
Graduate Center
City University of New York and Hunter College
New York, New York

Angela Northrup, MSN, RN, FNP
Clinical Assistant Professor
Pace University
College of Health Professions
Lienhard School of Nursing
Pleasantville, New York

Susan Salmond, EdD, RN, FAAN
Interim Dean
University of Medicine and Dentistry
School of Nursing
Newark, New Jersey

Joanne Singleton, PhD, RN, FNP-BC
Professor and Chairperson
Department of Graduate Studies
Pace University
College of Health Professions
Lienhard School of Nursing
New York, New York

Jason T. Slyer, DNP, RN, FNP-BC
Clinical Assistant Professor
Pace University
College of Health Professions
Lienhard School of Nursing
New York, New York

Andréa Sonenberg, PhD, WHNP, CNM-BC
Associate Professor
Pace University
College of Health Professions
Lienhard School of Nursing
Pleasantville, New York

Linda Berger Spivack, MS, RN, CENP
Statewide Directory
Connecticut Nursing Collaborative-Action Coalition
Meriden, Connecticut
Doctoral Student in PhD Nursing Program
Graduate Center at the City University of New York
New York, New York

Harry Jacobs Summers, JD
Senior Advisor
The Center for Nursing Advocacy
Baltimore, Maryland

Sandy Summers, RN, MSN, MPH
Executive Director
The Center for Nursing Advocacy
Baltimore, Maryland

Lorraine Von Eeden, DNP, CPNP
Pace University
New York, New York

Sharon Stahl Wexler, PhD, RN
Assistant Professor
Pace University
College of Health Professions
Lienhard School of Nursing
New York, New York

Chapter 1

Know Yourself: Reflective Decision-Making

Marie Truglio-Londrigan and
Sandra B. Lewenson

The genesis for this book was a graduate course in decision-making that we taught, titled "Advanced Decision-Making in Primary Health Care," which was one of the core courses in the graduate program at our school (O'Donnell, Lewenson, & Keith-Anderson, 2000). The course covered the various approaches to decision-making including self-reflection, history, economics, culture, family, evidence-based practice, media, group decision-making, and healthcare policy. These various approaches were to be used by nurses in all healthcare settings, but actual clinical decision-making tools were not part of this course. In preparing for the course, we found that no text existed that addressed the topics we covered. After searching the literature, the faculty developed a "course pack" that contained the course readings; eventually we placed our readings on the library electronic reserve.

This worked for several years, until faculty decided we wanted a more consistent way of sharing with our students and with a larger nursing audience what we had learned over time about decision-making. This required more than grouping the readings together and posting them. It required a way of translating and explaining to others what we meant by decision-making. This meant we needed to think through our thoughts on decision-making.

The changing landscape in nursing education calls for nurses at both the baccalaureate and graduate level to be leaders (American Association of Colleges of Nursing [AACN], 2008, 2011). Both the master's and baccalaureate essentials are laced with the term *leadership*, albeit at different levels. Based on their need to be leaders, both levels of students are asked to be reflective in their practice. Undergraduate students are asked to "Reflect on one's own beliefs and values as they relate to professional practice" (AACN, 2008, p. 29); graduate students are asked to be reflective practitioners with an emphasis on considering culturally competent practice: "Each practitioner should be engaged continuously in self reflection about their own personal beliefs, norms, behaviors and language and how together they guide their perceptions, beliefs, and interactions with patients" (AACN, 2008, p. 33). Nurses reflect on their decisions; understanding this approach to decision-making makes it imperative that we consider the idea of leadership as we consider the role self-reflection plays in nursing decisions.

Self-Reflection and Decision-Making

When making decisions, nurses need to understand that decision-making requires looking inward at one's own self, then outward at the world around them, and then back in again. The decision-making process requires us to understand that the particular issue that needs a decision can often become unfocused, very much like a holographic image. As this distortion becomes evident to the decision-maker (in this instance the nurse), it is important to recognize it for what it is and to scan the environment for knowledge that helps the nurse bring the image back into focus, which allows a decision to be made. The process of knowledge attainment may require a variety of approaches, including self-reflection, history, legal, ethical, spirituality, culture, family, group/team, evidence-based practice, economics, technology, and health policy, especially when one considers the knowledge, competencies, and skills that nurses and nursing leaders must hold and exemplify. In the first edition of this text we wanted to codify what we were teaching about decision-making in one text that could explain our ideas. The same holds true in this second edition with the expansion of ideas and decision-making approaches that are reflective of the wide variety of healthcare practice settings.

While writing this text, the coeditors spent a great deal of time discussing decision-making. We asked ourselves: What does decision-making mean? How can we approach it? How can we teach students and nurses to use various approaches and strategies in their decision-making? What have we learned from others? What is our own "brand" or philosophical thoughts about decision-making? Finally, we asked: How can we learn from ourselves? We both believe that in order to make meaningful decisions, a self-reflective process has to take place. Within a self-reflective process, one must examine one's own ideas, values, and beliefs. In addition, one must be able to "bracket" these beliefs (like in qualitative research) in search of answers or decisions that support care. Schön's work (1983), *The Reflective Practitioner: How Professionals Think in Action*, offers guidance in this regard. Schön identifies that health professionals frequently are holders of information and knowledge that is tacit and that "competent practitioners usually know more than they can say" (p. viii), or they exhibit a "kind of knowing-in-practice" (p. viii). How one comes to know what one knows or what one is about is through reflective practice (Coakley & Scoble, 2003; Schön, 1983).

Self-reflection becomes an integral part of the process that allows the decision-maker to be thoughtful in the approaches he or she uses in making decisions. There is an ebb and flow of ideas that create synergy between and among the various approaches to decision-making. The synergy provides an opportunity to examine the various factors that enter into decision-making—the looking inward, outward, and then in again described earlier. The ability to understand the choices one has when making decisions and the concomitant risks that one takes with the choices selected must also be considered during the decision-making process (Buchanan & O'Connell, 2006). Nursing leader Angela Barron McBride's (2011) text, *The Growth and Development of Nurse Leaders*, uses reflection throughout in her exploration of leadership. Using her own experiences she explores the personal and professional sides of leadership. She states that she wanted to write a text that was peppered with "personal reflections and scholarly references" (McBride, 2011, p. xv). In one example, McBride writes about how the story one tells oneself in a given situation will shape that person's reality; ultimately, the choices he or she makes about that reality play out in his or her decisions. Self-reflection, knowing who you are, is central to becoming and being a leader.

Self-reflection was defined by the course faculty "as an examination of one's own thoughts and feelings, [and] requires maturity and a desire to know who you are" (O'Donnell et al., 2000, p. 153). We used this definition with our students and recognized that the students, many of whom were enrolled in the family nurse practitioner program, were adult learners and therefore mature enough to examine who they were so that they could use their reflections on self to acquire and generate knowledge (Mountford & Rogers, 1996;

O'Donnell et al., 2000). More recently, this definition and the key points of self-reflection and the various decision-making models is being provided to a broader audience including nursing education students and our Doctoral of Nursing Practice students. Other healthcare disciplines, such as physical therapy, also consider the use of self-reflection in decisions. Based on their research, Wainwright, Shepard, Harman, & Stephens (2010) determined that "the development of these skills of reflection is necessary to take assessment and decision making in the clinical setting beyond textbook knowledge to patient management that recognizes the values, ethics, and preferences of the participants" (p. 84).

In this chapter we use ourselves to explain what we mean by self-reflection and how the self-reflective process bears on decision-making. We think that by doing this we demonstrate how self-reflection may impact on decisions we make in life and how this impacts the decisions we help others make. In class we used a similar type of exercise to help students reflect on their own selves and see how who they are impacts their decisions. In order to accomplish this goal, we introduce ourselves through self-reflection. We describe who we are, our backgrounds, and our education and relate how these experiences shaped our philosophy and the decisions we have made. We deviate from the *Publication Manual of the American Psychological Association* by using our first names and speaking from a personal perspective. We believe this provides the readers a more intimate connection with the editors of this book and is more in keeping with the language of self-reflection.

Use of Self

We learned throughout this project that we were similar in the way we looked at decision-making. First, we both knew that decision-making required a way of looking at the world that was synchronous with what we believed about nursing. We shared a holistic world view typically held by nurses, especially public health nurses (which we both are). For us, this meant that there was no one approach to use when making decisions. We both recognized that decision-making is a fluid process in which self-reflection, listening to others, knowledge of various frameworks, and ways of knowing (Carper, 1992) unfold simultaneously in a synergistic process that supports decision-making.

The way we make decisions is influenced by many intra- and interpersonal characteristics like our style, our culture, where we grew up, our education, our personality, and how we perceive the world. We both selected research methods that allowed for our world view or perspective to come through. For example, Marie's hermeneutical study, *The Unfolding Meaning of the Wisdom Experience*, explores the phenomenon of wisdom as it unfolds within the context of a nurse–patient relationship and the decision-making process that lies inherent in that experience (Truglio-Londrigan, 2002). The process that Marie uses for decision-making somewhat mirrors the process she used in the hermeneutical method. Gadamer's (1976) philosophical hermeneutical approach is based on the language of conversation, which provides a medium for understanding as individuals use language to express themselves and listen. This holds true with the decision-making process. Once conversation facilitates understanding via language and listening, the outcome is not only understanding, but also the ability to identify a decision and act on it. This dialogue, questioning, and conversation stand at the center of Gadamer's philosophical hermeneutics (Bernstein, 1983) and portrays an interplay. This interplay is that same looking inward and outward and then back inward again described earlier.

Sandy's world view is colored by the research that she does in nursing history. The antecedents to events, knowledge, therapeutic interventions, and the like all contribute to how she approaches decision-making. To her, decisions require an understanding of the historical antecedents. Historical research offers critique of an assortment of historical events, people, issues, therapeutic events, and the like, which offers insight into decision-making. For example, in a 2007 *New York Times* article, McNeil recommended federal guidelines to deal with a severe flu outbreak that were "partly based on a recent study of how 44 cities fared in the 1918 epidemic conducted jointly by the disease centers and the University of Michigan's medical school" (p. A14). In this study, it was the historians and epidemiologists who examined how cities managed during the 1918 flu pandemic. Wall and Keeling (2013) provide analysis of how disasters in the past, like the 1918 flu pandemic, the Galveston Hurricane in 1900, and the Alaska earthquake in 1964, offer insight into nursing care needed at these times of crisis. The past provided a way to analyze the possible ways of addressing a potential influenza epidemic today.

Know Yourself

How did we arrive at this juncture? How did we come to be here and think this way? In the following sections of this chapter, we will describe through our own self-reflective process how our philosophical beliefs about decision-making came to be, as well as our own comfort level with making a decision and accepting the risk involved in decision-making. When we make decisions, we each draw from our intra- and interperceptual experiences; however, without self-reflection and awareness of what the self brings to the decision-making process, decisions risk inadequacy or failure.

Marie's Self Reflection

I grew up in the Bronx, one of the five boroughs of New York City. There is no better place in the world, because in the Bronx I was introduced to life, in all its glory and sadness. My parents were high school graduates who worked hard day to day. My mother was a homemaker, my father a postal worker. Both parents were of Italian descent, although my father insisted that he was Sicilian; that was somehow different. My maternal grandmother and grandfather lived in the same apartment building as we did. My grandmother was 4 feet, 11 inches tall and packed a punch. My grandfather was 6 feet tall and an alcoholic. They were an integral part of our lives and were involved in my upbringing.

I was baptized Marie Truglio and welcomed into the Catholic church, although, as it turns out, I am much more of a spiritual being rather than a religious being. Life has always been one big question to me due to the various experiences I have been introduced to throughout my life.

When I was 3 years old, my sister was born. I remember sitting at my great aunt's kitchen table eating her wonderful pound cake in Queens, New York (another of the five boroughs) when there was a phone call. I remember that I did not know what they were saying, only that all of a sudden the atmosphere in the room changed. My great aunt looked at my father and said "Ann went into labor" to which my father responded, "How can that be? She's not at her due date." This single moment in time changed my life forever. My sister was born with a diagnosis of Down's syndrome. Everyone was so sad and yet I remember I could not understand why. She looked "okay" to me. It is true she did not do much, but is that not what all babies do, nothing? When I asked my parents why, they both said that my sister was sick. Sick? She did not appear sick. There never appeared to be any answers to those questions, but I have to say these life experiences created a context for me as being the "searcher": to raise questions and attempt to find answers—even if those answers were "correct" for only a moment in time.

I always asked questions. In the 1960s when riots were on the television every night, others would shake their heads and say "throw them all in jail," while I would question, "What is the reason for this? Why are these riots taking place? What can be done?" Similarly, when the news would account for the number of soldiers who died in Vietnam that day, again I would question, "Is this necessary? Who is right? What is the truth? Is there any truth at all?" My parents would listen to me rant on and on and never tell me to be quiet. They would just listen. This, I believe, was important. I always knew that I could say and do anything—within reason, of course—and I knew that I always would have my place in this family. I trusted, and this is the trust that is essential to make decisions.

I wanted to be a nurse because I thought I could help—help by stopping the riots, help by stopping the Vietnam War, or help by making my parents proud of something or someone. In any event, I made the decision that nursing was going to be my professional commitment. We wrote earlier about risk taking and the choices that we make in decision-making. Well, here was one. I was the first generation in my family to enter college in the United States. My grandmother had been a teacher in Italy, but when she came to this country she was told that she would never be a teacher here. She was not able to make a decision, the decision was made for her. I was frightened because I could not fail; therefore, I would not fail. I remember looking at my grandmother and thinking that I was an extension of her. I had to do this. Four years later, I graduated.

Since that time I have embarked on many decisions—some good and some not so good, like the white Volvo my husband and I bought from a car dump in New Jersey. Go figure! I can safely say that we did not use any type of evidence in this decision and it was a big risk and a big mistake, one from which we both learned. I should add that this, too, is important in decision-making: the importance of self-reflecting and learning from the outcomes of every decision no matter what they are. Nevertheless, other decisions were marked by successes—the decision to marry the man who continues as my husband, the decision to return to school for my master's degree, the decision to build our life and to include children within that life, and finally, the decision to engage in doctoral studies. Every decision portrayed a risk, but as I stated earlier, I trusted and this was the trust that my parents modeled for me. They would love me no matter what I said or what I did.

As I stated before, throughout my life, whenever I had to make a decision, I was a searcher. I first would look inward to see what was there. When I found that what I saw was distorted or unclear, I would look outward. Where could I go to find the answers that would clear up this distortion? Once I found what I thought I needed, I would take that knowledge and return to my inner self to see if the distortion was still present or if the picture was clear. There have been times, however, when clarity never was attained and I have since learned that sometimes one must live with unknowing. A diagnosis of breast cancer 5 years ago led me to the difficult decision of a bilateral mastectomy. It was amazing to me how in the acknowledgement of my own mortality a major shift occurred in my world view. At one point in my past life I was unable to live with uncertainty. Now, I can accept it and I recognize it as an unforeseen outcome of this event.

It permits me not to be so rigid and to be able to shift and change. It also helps me to be more open and aware of others and also accepting of differences. Ultimately, what I learned is that for any decision, the comfort of coming to a decision was always short lived. It only lasts for a moment in time because every moment brings newness—hence, my love for hermeneutics as well as the way I conduct myself and look at the world, one moment at a time. I believe Boyd and Fales (1983) stated it best: "Reflective learning is the process of internally examining and exploring an issue of concern triggered by an experience, which creates and clarifies meaning in terms of self, and which results in a changed conceptual perspective" (p. 99).

Sandy's Self-Reflection

I was born in 1949 and, like Marie, I too was born in the Bronx. I was the second of three daughters and one son. My parents also grew up in the Bronx, attended the same synagogue, and attended the same university in New York City.

My family was not the typical Jewish family. We were Reform Jews, with the roots of this progressive movement stemming back three generations to Germany. We did not grow up in a Jewish neighborhood because my parents wanted us to experience people from all different backgrounds. We lived in a multiethnic and multiracial community that was situated in the northeast section of the Bronx called Wakefield. There were homemade raviolis, a German butcher and deli, a kosher deli, a bakery run by Hungarian immigrants, and assorted other ethnic-type food stores that lined the streets under the subway's elevated or "El" pillars on White Plains Road.

My family did things that many of my friends on the block or in most other Bronx neighborhoods did not do. Every summer my parents packed the car, gave each one of us a cardboard box to hold our belongings, and off we went on a camping trip. We were often labeled "gypsies" by friends and family alike because for most of the summer we lived in a tent. My parents started their own hand-guided quilting business, even without having much knowledge about this type of business, and were deeply involved with local Bronx politics—so much so that my father would recruit the whole family (including some of my dates) to hang the candidates' posters on the subway elevator track poles that lined the avenue near our home.

Both sets of grandparents were born in the United States, which was unusual at the time, at least in our neighborhood. My father's parents died before I was born, so I never met them, but I heard about them, especially about how my grandmother, Lillian Nibur, was a teacher and a suffragist. My mother's grandparents, Monroe and Jennie, were both born in the United States but never completed high school; however, they always valued education. It was no surprise to me growing up that I was going to go to college. We saw Monroe and Jennie every Saturday and they played a prominent role in our family's day-to-day life.

When I was 12, my younger sister, who was 7 at the time, died of cystic fibrosis. At that time, little was known about this disease. The cost of care was too high for our family so my father had to find a job in New York City that afforded us health insurance and access to care. He also drove a cab at night to "make ends meet," as my mother would often say. From my memory, we were one of the first families to enroll in the newly formed Health Insurance Plan (HIP) at Montefiore Hospital in the Bronx in about 1962. I remember hearing how the doctors and nurses were trying new treatments for this disease and my sister was given antibiotics, cupping, and other exercises to help her breathe better. In the summer after my sister died, we left for a camping trip across the United States. No matter what had happened that previous year, we kept exploring new environments, new places, and new ideas. One of my father's favorite expressions was "to try it."

Growing up, I loved music, color, dance, and anything that allowed me to move. Today, I probably would be labeled a "kinetic" learner, but in the 1950s and 1960s, learning was mostly done sitting down. My decision to become a nurse probably stemmed from the experience I had with my sister growing up and my need to move. When I decided to become a nurse, my parents were not happy with that decision and tried to steer me toward teaching. They felt nursing was not the right profession to be in, whether because of the images they held about the profession (and that was never clear to me) or because they felt teaching was easier for women who wanted a family. In any event, they agreed with my decision to become a nurse but with the caveat that I attend a collegiate program, not a diploma school. Education was important in my family, and thus shaped my decision about becoming a baccalaureate-prepared nurse.

I met my husband while in nursing school. He attended the dental school a few blocks away. We both marched during the 1960s and early 1970s protests against the Vietnam War, served as health workers at some of the stations that were set up around the city to assist the marchers, and shared many of the same hopes for a country that was undergoing changes in civil rights, women's rights, and healthcare reforms. My husband was born in Rosenheim, Germany, following World War II. I include this piece of history because our two families, both Jewish, both in a healthcare profession, were so diverse in our cultural backgrounds that decisions we made as a family required real consensus building and an understanding of cultural backgrounds.

My love of history stemmed from my need to understand and explain the world. Growing up, I needed to know. I did not understand the reasons for so many things and always sought answers.

My older sister was labeled the "smart one"; my brother was the "man-child"; my sister who died held a special place in the family system because of her illness; I was the middle one and took up the mantle of being the "clown." I could imitate any one of my many teachers, tell jokes, and generally entertained my family on a nightly basis. The humor was my way of knowing and explaining the world.

I did not become interested in nursing history until I returned to school for a master's degree more than 10 years following my graduation from my baccalaureate program. Following the completion of a quantitative master's thesis on determining the market for the independent practice of a family nurse clinician, I became increasingly aware that most people did not know that nurses went to college, never mind graduate school. It was not until my doctoral work that I learned to use historical method as a way of understanding why most people had no idea about what nursing was or how one became educated as a nurse. It was raising questions and being ready to explore the historical data to find answers that helped me make the decision to study nursing history. Historical research helped me understand the things that I could no longer laugh about, like why nurses were not valued (perhaps a remnant of the way my family responded to my being a nurse) or why we do not remember nursing's political activity . . . or that they were even political or ever involved. (I always remembered the noted public health nurse Lillian Wald and related her to the progressive movement, but somehow that knowledge was not included in my daughter's social studies textbook, which described Wald as a social worker.)

Understanding my background helps me to understand why I made certain decisions about my education, my practice, my research, and my professional goals. It continues to influence me as I make other decisions in life. There are many choices—and many risks. How and what we choose is indicative of our ability to be self-reflective and to understand and generate knowledge. How we, as nursing professionals, help others make decisions also is influenced by our backgrounds. Being self-reflective and understanding who we are is essential to the decision-making process.

Self-Reflection Assists Decision-Making

Both of us were born in the Bronx in New York City and both are part of the baby boomer population that exploded following World War II. Both of our fathers served in World War II. Both of us had sisters who had health-related issues that left indelible marks. We both grew up in family systems where grandparents were involved and education was important. Our educational experiences were different because Marie went to Catholic school and Sandy went to Bronx public schools. In terms of religion, Marie would classify her family as deeply rooted in the practice of Catholicism, whereas Sandy's family espoused the more liberal attitudes of Reform Judaism. We each chose a 4-year baccalaureate degree in nursing because college education was highly valued in our families. Even our choice of clinical setting, public health nursing, was similar because Sandy enjoyed being outside and moving, and Marie felt there was a potential to make an impact for the greater good. We both agree that there was greater autonomy and freedom to choose in this setting than in others. Serendipity brought us together to work at the same institution, teach the same course, and write this book, but it was also our backgrounds and the knowledge we gained from being self-reflective that led us to this point.

The decisions we make and the ones we help others make in our practice all have some elements of our past interacting with the decision, whether consciously or unconsciously. This, then, makes it imperative for all of us who are in a healthcare profession to be aware of what we consider worthwhile, such as a special treatment, the healthcare provider we visit, the hospital we select, or the treatment plan we follow. Do we exercise to stay healthy, or avoid any kind of health-promoting or preventative-type activities? Do we smoke or do we have difficulty watching anyone who does? What are our values related to health care, and how do our biases affect the very people we are caring for? The practice of self-reflection, then, becomes essential to any decisions that nurses make.

In this chapter we wanted to introduce ourselves and, through self-reflection, demonstrate how past life experience affects how we live in the world, how we perceive the world, and how we conduct ourselves when making decisions. To us, decision-making is more than a model or framework—it is a philosophy intimately intertwined with our view of the world. Self-reflection creates awareness and knowledge building. It also helped us formulate our philosophy about decision-making. Our histories share many similarities and differences, and the decisions we make and help others make reflect this.

It is clear to us that how we engage in the decision-making process has more to do with philosophy than any one approach to decision-making. This philosophy has unfolded over the years as a result of life experiences. Self-reflection allows us access to this knowledge and gives a clearer picture of ourselves, so that we can ultimately use this knowledge when we make decisions and help the various constituents in our practice make their decisions. Self-reflection serves as an integral part of the decision-making process for all nurses. An awareness of who we are opens us up to the possibility of who others may be and how we interact with them in therapeutic relationships. Reflective decision-making requires self-reflection using a variety of thoughtful approaches.

References

American Association of Colleges of Nursing (AACN) (2008). *The essentials of baccalaureate education for professional nursing practice*. Retrieved from http://www.aacn.nche.edu/education-resources/essential-series

American Association of Colleges of Nursing (AACN) (2011). *The essentials of master's education in nursing*. Retrieved from http://www.aacn.nche.edu/education-resources/essential-series

Bernstein, R. (1983). *Beyond objectivism and relativism: Science, hermeneutics, and praxis*. Philadelphia: University of Pennsylvania Press.

Boyd, E., & Fales, A. (1983). Reflective learning: Key to learning from experience. *Journal of Humanistic Psychology, 23*(2), 99–117.

Buchanan, L., & O'Connell, A. (2006). A brief history of decision-making. *Harvard Business Review, 84*(1), 32–37.

Carper, B. A. (1992). Philosophical inquiry in nursing: An application. In J. E. Kikuchi & H. Simmons (Eds.), *Philosophical inquiry in nursing* (pp. 71–80). London: Sage Publications.

Coakley, E., & Scoble, K. B. (2003). A reflective model for organizational assessment and interventions. *Journal of Nursing Administration, 33*(12), 660–669.

Gadamer, H. G. (1976). *Philosophical hermeneutics* (D. Ling, Trans. & Ed.). Los Angeles, CA: University of California Press.

McBride, A. B. (2011). *The growth and development of nurse leaders*. New York: Springer Publishing Company.

McNeil, D. G. (2007, February 7). Closings and cancellations top advice on flu outbreak. *The New York Times*, p. A14.

Mountford, B., & Rogers, L. (1996). Using individual and group reflection in and on assessment as a tool for effective learning. *Journal of Advanced Nursing, 24*, 1127–1134.

O'Donnell, J. P., Lewenson, S. B., & Keith-Anderson, K. (2000). Who am I?: Teaching nurse practitioner students to develop self-reflective practice. In M. K. Crabtree (Ed.), *Teaching clinical decision-making in advanced nursing practice*, pp. 153–159. Washington, DC: National Organization of Nurse Practitioner Faculties.

Schön, D. A. (1983). *The reflective practitioner: How professionals think in action*. New York: Basic Books.

Truglio-Londrigan, M. (2002). An analysis of wisdom: An experience in nursing practice. *Journal of the New York State Nurses Association, 33*(2), 24–30.

Wainwright, S. F., Shepard, K. F., Harman, L. B., & Stephens, J. (2010). Novice and experienced physical therapist clinicians: A comparison of how reflection is used to inform the clinical decision-making process. *Physical Therapy, 90*(1), 75–89.

Wall, B. M., & Keeling, A. (2013). Historical highlights in disaster nursing. In M. Truglio-Londrigan and S. B. Lewenson. *Public health nursing: Practicing population-based care* (2nd ed). (pp. 353–367), Burlington, MA: Jones & Bartlett.

Chapter 2

Looking Back: History and Decision-Making in Health Care

Sandra B. Lewenson

Nurses make decisions every day that affect the health of the individuals, families, communities, and populations they serve. They make decisions about the use of clinical interventions, the use of their political vote, the education of nurses, the application of new technologies, and a myriad of other issues as well—yet when nurses make decisions, they often use decision-making frameworks that do not take into account past practices. Nelson and Gordon (2004) write about the "rhetoric of rupture," stating that nurses often discard and distance themselves from their past, leaving huge gaps in their knowledge. Nurses continually reinvent themselves and their practice at the expense of their history. Without understanding and valuing past contributions to practice or to society, nurses contribute to the "nursism" or bias toward the caring role that pervades this society (Lewenson, 1993). The omission of what nurses do on a day-to-day basis is a loss for both current and future generations of nurses and to others who might benefit from such knowledge.

In 1939, nurse historian Mary Roberts wrote that the "trends and events of today are the results of past experience as well as of varying conceptions of both present and future needs" (p. 1). Roberts recognized the need to examine the history of nursing to see how the profession could move forward. Another nurse historian, Teresa Christy (1978), explained how she could not "emphasize enough the relevance of an understanding of yesterday's problems for illumination of today's issues and concomitant potential for tomorrow's solutions" (p. 5). More recently, historians Patricia D'Antonio and Julie Fairman (2010) wrote, "History provides a critically important perspective if we are to understand and address contemporary health system problems" (p. 113). The historical perspective and context of a particular issue can help in the decision-making of healthcare policies and nursing practice. D'Antonio and Fairman (2010) further explain that

> ... issues of quality and safety, for example, are not new: they led directly to the formation of training schools in hospitals throughout the country in the late 19th century as physicians needed what we have called in other work "educated allies" to maintain asepsis in surgical suites and on hospital wards. (p. 113)

And later Fairman and D'Antonio (2013) write, "historical influence can be subtle, difficult to extract, and contradictory, but its impact can be far-reaching and enduring" (p. 346). Regardless of whether nurses choose to use history in their decision-making process, history impacts their decisions. Keeling and Lewenson (2013) further note that history not only impacts decisions, but influences health policy, such as how society views issues addressing who should lead medical homes. Thus, as part of a reflective decision-making process, nurses need to know and value their history to make meaningful decisions about their current and future work. This chapter explores why history helps nurses in their decision-making process as well as briefly describes the history of decision-making in nursing.

Historical research provides a way of understanding the past and therefore provides a framework in which to study and apply history to decision-making. Although it is beyond the scope of this chapter to discuss the steps used in historical research, it identifies some of the historical studies that contribute to the evidence used in practice and professional growth. The case study opening this chapter illustrates how graduate nursing students use historical evidence to support the decision-making process in a community health clinical experience. The historical research presented later in this chapter offers examples of how history informs the decision-making efforts and thus enhances the leadership skills required by nurses when making decisions. The case study closing this chapter provides an illustration of how historical knowledge about nursing roles would help current nurses in their practice.

Case Study

A Community Assessment of the Lower East Side of New York City, 1893

What began as a study to look at the Lower East Side of New York City as Lillian Wald may have seen it when she established the Henry Street Settlement became an exciting exercise for contemporary students to explore how decisions were made. Nurses need to be able to assess a community and determine the types of services that would most benefit the community. To teach nurses how to assess a community, prioritize the community's primary health care needs, plan and develop an appropriate intervention, and examine the impact of their decisions, historical data were used. In this case study, graduate nursing students interested in community and the Henry Street Settlement in the Lower East Side of New York City joined in doing a historical community assessment as part of their requirement for a master's project. To complete this requirement, they examined the period of time in which the Henry Street Settlement house was first organized.

The Henry Street Settlement was started in 1893 by two public health nurses, Lillian Wald and her friend, Mary Brewster. Using the demographic data, photographs, and selected writings from 1893 enabled the current students to more fully understand what Wald and Brewster might have seen when they first established the nurses' settlement house on the Lower East Side of New York. The study helped students learn why Wald and Brewster opened a nurses' settlement house in the area, the kinds of healthcare issues they found, and the impact that their nursing decisions had on the health of that community. In addition, this project enabled students to look at the professional and healthcare issues over time and see how they compared with those of today. They used history to help them understand the role of the visiting nurse, the political activism that the nurses exhibited, and the obligation to society that nurses continue to maintain now in the twenty-first century. They also used their findings to help them make decisions about community health initiatives in the same community more than 100 years later.

Students studied the Lower East Side community, specifically the area designated as the seventh and tenth wards. In the late nineteenth century, New York City was divided into wards rather than the present-day census tracts, and data were therefore collected according to ward and sanitary districts. The students examined the demographics; morbidity and mortality rates; immigration patterns; police, fire, and sanitation support services; educational, religious, and social institutions in the community; and political and nursing issues of that period. Students identified the priority needs in the community and compared their ideas with the actual contributions of the nurses at Henry Street. The students learned about the overcrowded living conditions that so many of the immigrants who populated the Lower East Side found in the tenements. In 1893 the total population in Manhattan (a borough of New York City in which the Lower East Side was a small section) totaled 1,758,000. About 1,332,773, or 69 percent of the total population, lived in the tenements of the Lower East Side. There were 180,359 children under the age of 5 (New York Board of Health, 1909).

The data showed that the residents of the Lower East Side came from Italy, Germany, Hungary, Russia, and other European countries. Once they arrived in the United States and moved to the Lower East Side, they found the tenements waiting for them. They experienced six-floor walk-up apartments, a lack of running water (this was prior to the cold-water flats that evolved following the inclusion of sinks in the tenements), outdoor plumbing until plumbing moved onto the hallway of each floor, as well as poor ventilation and poor lighting. Families, regardless of their size, resided in the two rooms that made up the apartments of the early tenements. Lack of privacy was just one of the many insults to the human condition that existed for those who lived in the tenements. The Tenement Museum in New York shows what life in the tenements was like, and students were able to access the museum's Web site (www.tenement.org) as well as personally visit this setting.

The inadequate housing conditions as well as the inhumane work conditions of so many of the immigrants contributed to the poor health conditions that they experienced. Some of the findings showed that infants accounted for 25 percent of all deaths in the community and that children under 5 accounted for 40 percent of all deaths in the community. The top causes of death in 1893 were pneumonia, phthis (pulmonary tuberculosis), digestive organ diseases, heart disease, and diphtheria. Infectious diseases were the cause of 42 percent of the deaths in this community, with pneumonia, phthis, diarrhea, and diphtheria leading the list of these illnesses (New York Board of Health, 1897, 1909).

Students learned that between 1892 and 1893 there was a 30 percent increase in suicide and that immigrants accounted for 80 percent of these suicides. They further examined how the social, economic, and political factors occurring around 1893 may have affected the suicide rates among the immigrant population. The financial depression of 1893 in the United States surely may have contributed to the increase in the number of suicides during this period. Students explored crime statistics and literacy rates, as well as houses of worship, social services, and other important areas of community support. They could visualize the effects of—or lack of—these supports by the outcomes they observed in the morbidity and mortality rates (New York Board of Health, 1897).

Students also read some of Wald's writings and began to learn about the programs that Wald and Brewster, along with the Henry Street nurses, brought to the community. The Henry Street visiting nurses, the students learned, lived at the settlement house and became neighbors of the families they served. They read about Wald's famous "baptism by fire": she met a young child who led her through the streets of the Lower East Side to visit her mother, who had been hemorrhaging for 2 days in bed after a difficult childbirth. Wald's graphic description provides a stark reality that allowed students to relate to the experience. Wald (1915) wrote:

> Through Hester and Division streets we went to the end of Ludlow; past odorous fish-stands, for the streets were a marketplace, unregulated, unsupervised, unclean; past evil-smelling, uncovered garbage-cans; and—perhaps worst of all, where so many little children played. . . . The child led me on through a tenement hallway, across a court where open and unscreened closets were promiscuously used by men and women, up into a rear tenement, by slimy steps whose accumulated dirt was augmented that day by the mud of the streets, and finally into the sickroom. . . . Although the family of seven shared their two rooms with boarders . . . and although the sick woman lay on a wretched, unclean bed, soiled with a hemorrhage two days old, they were not degraded human beings . . . that morning's experience was a baptism of fire." (pp. 5–6)

Soon after Wald met the family of seven, she and her friend, Mary Brewster, began the Henry Street Settlement for the express purpose of improving the unhealthy living conditions they found in the community. Both nurses were social activists and strove to improve the life of the residents of the Lower East Side through political action and nursing interventions. Wald, especially, felt that nurses had the knowledge and skills to advocate political changes to improve the health of the families in the community. Wald (1900/1991) explained that

> ... among the many opportunities for civic and altruistic work pressing on all sides nurses having superior advantages in their practical training should not rest content with being only nurses, but should use their talents wherever possible in reform and civic movements. (p. 318)

Wald's belief that nurses were poised to advocate for change in the social, economic, and political conditions of the community in which they lived led to many of the reforms that contributed to the health of the citizens in the community. For example, Wald visited families in their home, providing access to nursing care; organized well-baby classes for new mothers; advocated the first school nurse program in New York City, which placed a nurse in a city school; established a playground in the community, one of the first of its kind; and fostered an intellectual community of nurses who actively lobbied for social and political changes that supported the health of the citizens in the community.

Given the data that the students collected in their community assessment, they felt there was synergy between the programs that Wald established and the data they collected. Through the data, they witnessed the sights that Wald and Brewster saw as they made decisions to provide primary health care in the community. Students also saw the similarities between 1893 and the twenty-first century. What seemed to exist in 1893 continues to exist in a different (but similar) form. The inability to gain access to affordable care due to lack of sufficient funds or health insurance options, a rise in tuberculosis, women as primary caregivers, a close relationship between poverty and, large groups of immigrant populations, the need for social and political activism to support healthcare initiatives, and environmental factors affecting the health of children and adults in the community continue to be concerns in the same community in the twenty-first century. Students saw how public health nurses became leaders in health care because of the decisions they made. Although variations exist today on the particular environmental concerns, patterns of immigration, and political climate, what continues to be a constant is the need for nurses to make decisions about care and provide leadership in improving the health of individuals, families, and the communities they serve.

The students' use of history to learn about community assessments, community action, and nursing's role in political activism helped decide the kinds of health-promoting interventions they could use in their own community clinical experience. Understanding the history of Henry Street offers a way for students to see how decisions were made in the past and to value the remarkable outcomes that these decisions rendered in the nursing profession and the health of the community. They used some of the ideas of the past and introduced them with the ideas that they learned about primary health care in the twenty-first century. Teaching parenting skills, like Wald did in 1893, was one of the projects students initiated at Henry Street's abused women's shelter. Classes in parenting, nutrition, and other health promotion–type activities, which reflected the current thinking of the nursing students, continued the kinds of programming that the original public health nurses of the settlement house offered to the community. Students also saw the leadership displayed by Wald and other public health nurses in the late nineteenth and early twentieth centuries and how their activism continued to be a model for nurses today.

Nursing History Informs the Decision-Making Process

History provides a knowledge base that allows nurses to better understand their practice and profession. Knowing the evolution of nursing care, or the reasons why nurses for almost 100 years have debated the educational level into practice, or why each state requires separate licensing of nursing professionals affords nurses a way to understand the challenges that the profession has faced over time. Historical understanding allows for thoughtful decisions that facilitate innovation and change. Sometimes, however, tradition is mistaken for historical knowledge and, thus, confounds the decision-making process. Pape (2003) states that an organization's valuing of tradition may cause it to oppose changes in practice. Although tradition is part of history, understanding the origins of tradition through historical research allows a basis for comparison, critique, and ultimately decisions that allow for change. Historical research, rather than tradition, should be the key element used in providing evidence to support the decision-making efforts of nursing professionals.

Historical evidence provides depth, perspective, and context to issues nurses face today; as a result, the American Association for the History of Nursing (AAHN) supports the inclusion of nursing history in the curriculum. Keeling (2001) writes in an AAHN position paper that "nurses in the 21st century will need more than sheer information; they will need a greater sensitivity to contextual variables and ambiguity if they are to critically evaluate the information they receive." Nurses need the ability to study, understand, and value history. Integrating nursing history into nursing curricula at all levels is essential to help nurses identify their history; obtain the necessary skills to explore, study, and understand their history; and ultimately to use history in their decision-making process (Keeling, 2001; Lewenson, 2004).

Studying history provides nurses a conceptualization of the modern nursing movement from 1873 to the present day and affords continuity between the past and present. This continuity allows nurses to avoid the familiar adage: "Those who do not study history are doomed to repeat it." For nurses, not using history in the decision-making process may waste valuable time and resources in reinventing what was already previously discovered to work (or not work). Not using history also may deny the success of decisions made in nursing education, practice, research, or administration. Nurses need to know what worked and what did not work, and how they can seek the data to support decisions that need to be made by nurses. History is a valuable resource as a knowledge base and can be used as a form of evidence. The graduate students in the Henry Street case study "saw" the conditions the newly immigrated families experienced in 1893 and some of the primary health care needs that Wald and her colleagues met. Without understanding the historical significance of the Lower East Side, the graduate students would miss the origins of some of the socially minded programs and ideology of the settlement houses that continue to exist in this area today. As students develop their historical knowledge, they are better able to situate some of the current issues being debated in the public arena, such as access to affordable care, into the decisions that are being made at the bedside as well as the national level.

Strumpf and Tomes (1993) examined the historical use of restraints in "troublesome patients" in the United States during the nineteenth century. They observed a difference between the common use of restraints in the United States versus the infrequent use of such devices in Great Britain. The cultural beliefs about the kind of care that these patients, including the mentally ill and the elderly, received differed historically in both countries and the outcomes of care varied as well. Strumpf and Tomes recognized the need to study history so that nurse administrators and nurses could examine their decisions about the use of restraints and gain a better understanding of why they continue to use them with the elderly when evidence does not support the use of these devices.

> Contemporary observers often assume that this modern restraint crisis is a peculiar product of the late twentieth century, with its large population of aged and chronically ill, fiscal crisis, institutional overcrowding, and staff turnover. . . . Many of the contemporary dilemmas involving physical restraint can be traced back to an earlier "restraint crisis" that occurred during the middle of the nineteenth century. (Strumpf & Tomes, 1993, p. 4)

Like Strumpf and Tomes, historians search for reasons why things occurred and do so in the hope of informing contemporary issues that need thoughtful decisions. When nurses do a nursing assessment on a patient, they start with a nursing history. Nurses would not be able to appropriately assess their patients or develop plans of action without one. If that is the case, why would nursing leaders, educators, practitioners, researchers, and the like attempt to make decisions without getting the history first?

A Historical Look at Decision-Making in Nursing

In exploring the use of nursing history in decision-making, it is important to look at the history of decision-making in nursing, or when and how nurses made decisions. Questions arise such as whether nurses actually made decisions overtly or just "downplayed" their own reasoning abilities to avoid alienating physicians if they assumed a more autonomous role. Did nurses always make decisions about care and about the profession? If so, what kinds of evidence did they use to make these decisions? How did they document these decisions? How did they take into account the lives of those they cared for, the political, social, or gendered roles that were prevalent at the time of study, or even now? Where was care situated—in the home, the office, or the hospital—and what did that mean for the care and the caregivers? How did nursing's close ties with the women's movement in the late 1800s and early 1900s affect the way nurses made decisions? Were nurses afraid of alienating politicians who could possibly help the nursing profession obtain nursing registration laws, as Lewenson (1993) suggests, or did they speak out in favor of women's suffrage, regardless of how it affected these politicians? Did Wald and Brewster use the same available demographic data as in the case study about the Lower East Side when determining the need for healthcare programs in the community? Have nurses historically used "evidence" to support their practice? If so, what kind of evidence did they use and how did they find the evidence?

Nursing research, important to the decision-making process, evolved in the profession as nursing educators and leaders called for nurses to base their clinical decisions on empirical evidence. Nursing educator R. Louise McManus (1961) asked the question, "What is the place of nursing research—yesterday, today, and tomorrow?" (p. 76), and examined the evolution of nursing research. She understood the need to look at how research influenced the decisions of nursing leaders in order to plan for the future in nursing. McManus explained that nursing research—or the "methodological search for nursing knowledge"—differed from that of other professional groups because early studies focused more on nursing education and service rather than on practice. She reasoned that interest in nursing research differed from other professions because of the different "pressures upon the profession as a whole by social, political, and economic forces and the impact on nursing advances in scientific knowledge" (p. 76).

McManus (1961) highlights the early research efforts of Florence Nightingale, and the later studies of M. Adelaide Nutting, Isabel Stewart, and others who examined nursing education and the status of the profession. The studies, McManus said, usually were implemented by professional organizations, like the American Society of Superintendents of Training Schools for Nurses (which was renamed the National League of Nursing Education in 1912, and then the National League for Nursing in 1952), and as a result focused more on the issues related to education. Nurse educators, like Stewart, valued research and participated in and led many such endeavors, such as her noted time-and-motion studies. Another noted nursing leader, Virginia Henderson, published early scientific studies such as the one McManus includes on "Medical and Surgical Asepsis" in 1939. Structure studies of how the professional organizations should look also were done and dramatically influenced the change in nursing organizations in the early 1950s.

McManus's (1961) examination of history provides a view of the development of nursing research prior to the early 1960s that explains as well as raises questions about nursing's interest in research and the subsequent culture of research. She noted that the way nursing organized around issues of practice and service as well as one of the first graduate educational programs for nurses situated in Teachers College, Columbia University (a college for teachers), was indicative of the kinds of studies and research of early nursing. McManus (1961) wrote that: "This happenstance of teachers pushing toward education and toward a teacher training institution for the first graduate programs may well have affected the course of nursing's development considerably" (p. 79).

Many in nursing were interested in knowledge building to support decisions in nursing. In her 1934 article in the *American Journal of Nursing*, Sister M. Bernice Beck called for nurses to base their practice on scientific principles rather than on outdated models that supported a paternalistic hierarchy. Nurses, especially educators and administrators, needed to have a "scientific attitude," which Beck described as being

> . . . openminded, ready to learn the truth and accept it; observant, keen, clear-minded, cautious, alert, vigorous, original, and independent in thinking; she carefully weighs all the evidence and overlooks no factor which may influence the results; allows no personal preferences to influence decisions; holds only tentative scientific convictions, because aware that we have not yet arrived at the end of knowledge, but are constantly wresting more secrets from the hidden depths of Nature." (p. 580)

The early move toward basing practice on nursing research required that nurses examine the way they carried out procedures and not just accept what they did without first examining the outcomes of their actions. Beck (1934) wrote that the teacher of nursing arts

> ... never insists that procedures, as taught, are the last word; that the unfounded statements of textbooks must be accepted without question, and that the ordering physician must be looked upon as an infallible authority. On the contrary, she urges her

> students to find out why things are done as they are; whether there are not better ways of doing them; to challenge statements, to ask for proofs, to think for themselves, to make individual contributions. (p. 581)

Students were expected to learn to question and to make decisions based on the response to their questions. Decisions were not to be made by rote; rather they needed to be made using research data. In their noted text, *The Principles and Practice of Nursing*, Harmer and Henderson (1940) included a section on the "Professional Responsibilities in Relation to Method." Nurses were to "accept the responsibility for studying its procedures and designing its method" (p. 469).

By the 1960s, educators like Francis Reiter (1966) advocated the use of basic sciences to govern the kind of care patients required and the use of rationale that directed the care she was providing. Reiter conceived of a master's prepared nurse who would be competent in three areas, namely, "ranges of function, depth of understanding, and breadth of services" (p. 274). Being clinically competent meant that nurses worked in an interdisciplinary collaboration with physicians, and like the physicians would be able to make decisions about patient care within the realm of nursing. Fairman's (2008) research on the development of nursing scholarship following World War II includes nurse educators like Reiter and others as they created clinical knowledge based on practice and research. As future generations of nursing scholars expanded on the ideas of these earlier educators, nursing decisions increasingly depended on research findings, rooting nursing practice within a scientifically oriented framework. Knowledge is contextual and contingent on the events of the day, and as such decisions nurses have made and will make must also be viewed within the context of the period in which they are made as well as the contingencies that affect these decisions.

In order to understand how decisions in nursing are made and the kinds of decision-making models or frameworks available, it is important to remember to place decisions within a context that looks at the particular period in which those decisions are made. The students in the case study presented earlier in this chapter examined the demographic data and the morbidity and mortality rates of the Lower East Side within the context of the late nineteenth-century United States. They explored the meaning of immigration within the social, political, and economic period of the day. In this way, they could compare and contrast the healthcare decisions that were made by nurses during that period with the more contemporary decisions made today in the same community. This may be beyond the scope of this chapter, but it is something to consider when looking at history and decision-making in nursing.

Historical Critiques Assist Decision-Making in Nursing

Historical research provides the data and the necessary critique that nurses require in their decision-making process. Historical evidence also provides a "sense of identity" and the tools to think critically when caring for others (Lewenson, 2013; Madsen, 2008, p. 525; Toman & Thifault, 2012). D'Antonio and Lewenson (2011) show how historical studies provide evidence for practice, earning "an important place in current practice" (p. xvi). For example, studies like the one by Arlene W. Keeling (2011) illustrate the work that nursing did during the 1918 influenza pandemic and has strong implications for nursing interventions today. Keeling's work, "Treating Influenza 1918 and 2010: Recycled Interventions," shows how strategies used in 1918 such as "advising patients to stay home, rest, and drink fluids until the flu subsided; to cover coughs and sneezes, to wash hands and to wear masks in public places" (p. 31) were not too different from the nursing interventions used today. Keeling (2011) wrote, "In fact, almost a century after the Great Flu of 1918, and despite major changes in medical and nursing therapeutics—including the availability of H1N1 vaccines and antiviral medications—much of the national and community response to the epidemic has been reminiscent of 1918" (p. 32). Keeling's analysis provides current healthcare providers, nurses in particular, an opportunity to understand the interventions that were used, as well as how these strategies were implemented. History provides depth and breadth to the decisions that are being made today when flu-like epidemics threaten the health and well-being of society.

A study by Cynthia Connolly (2011), "Determining Children's 'Best Interests' in the Midst of an Epidemic: A Cautionary Tale from History," uses nurses and the preventorium, an early twentieth-century institution designed to prevent the emergence of active tuberculosis in poor children who had tested positive to the newly developed tuberculin test, as a case study with which to explore the way society responds to the care of children. Connolly used the Farmingdale Tuberculosis Preventorium for Children, opened in 1909, to illustrate the issues surrounding the care of children who were diagnosed as "pretubercular" by the newly developed tuberculin test. The tuberculin test spawned a public health movement that hoped to save children before any symptoms of the disease appeared. An outcome of this public health initiative was the preventoria that opened throughout the United States. Children, typically from poor homes, who received this pretubercular diagnosis were removed from their homes and placed within one of these institutions. The preventoria, primarily run by nurses, were designed to reduce the progression of the dreaded disease. It was believed that poor children needed not only the kinds of interventions available at the time, such as light, good food, and rest, but also, as Connolly (2011) points out, "exposure to the social conditions and moral climate of the wealthier classes, treatment that was to be supplied through the institution's nurses" (p. 24). Connolly's analysis reflects on the care that these nurses provided, the interdisciplinary nature of their work with other healthcare providers who also shared the same goal in preventing tuberculosis, and the influence they had on healthcare policy and vice versa. Her study considers the tension among medical advances, the rights of the public, and the rights of families and children. The response to the epidemic was determined not only by the advances in science, but also by the ethnically, racially, and class-based bias that existed and influenced policies and the enactment of those policies. Connolly's research offers nurses and other healthcare providers insights into the kinds of decisions that are being made as we address other kinds of epidemics in children today, such as obesity. What decisions are being made and what the reasoning is behind these decisions must be considered. Nursing leaders can use Connolly's research to explore issues about the strategies being used in the care of children today, specifically poorer children.

Rima Apple's (2011) study, "To Avoid Expense and Suffering: Public Health Nurses and the Struggle for Health Services," opens with a description of a recent program called the Nurse-Family Partnership Program that provides evidence-based care to new mothers considered high risk. These women are assigned a nurse who makes home visits for a 2-year period starting prior to the birth of the infant. Apple compares the description of this program to one that existed 70 years prior in Wisconsin, called the Wisconsin Bureau of Maternal and Child Health (MCH). In a description of this earlier program, the director wrote that a public health nurse could visit expectant mothers and infants, provide health education in the homes of these families, and by doing so, improve the health of these mothers and infants. Although 70 years may have separated these two organizations, they shared a similar goal. The MCH, however, had even greater goals than simply providing care—it also advocated for local governmental support of a public health program that sent nurses into the homes of this population.

Apple's study explored the essential role that nurses have played and continue to play in public health initiatives such as this one, especially in rural America. In this study, Apple looks at the high infant and maternal mortality rates in the early twentieth century and their effect on the health of the nation. Families living in rural settings, in particular, needed access to health care and health education programs. Although some programs were available in rural Wisconsin, such as the

Well-Child Trailers in the 1920s, limitations to this care existed, such as lack of continuity of care, lack of access to medical care, and lack of understanding of what the conditions in the home were like. As a result, the MCH staff argued the case for a public health nurse to be assigned to each county of the state in order to provide the care that was needed to the families in those counties.

Apple (2011) used a case study of Barron County, Wisconsin, during the 1930s and the work of two MCH demonstration nurses to show the "complicated role that demonstration nurses played to effect the establishment and maintenance of a critical public health initiative" (p. 177). The Bureau of Public Health sent Louise Steffen, a nurse from Milwaukee who earned a certificate in public health nursing from Marquette University in Milwaukee, to become Barron County's first district MCH demonstration nurse in 1940. Apple studied Steffen's description of her work and the frustrations she encountered when dealing with the conditions she found in this rural county. Travel for her, like for the mothers she visited, was made difficult by the long distances on poor roads that existed between physicians, healthcare centers, and patients' homes. A heavy workload, unhelpful physicians, and inaccessible roads created challenges for Steffen as she continued to develop the role of public health nurse in the county in hopes of convincing the county to hire a full-time public health nurse, one of the aims of the demonstration project that sent her to this area. Her frustration with the difficult conditions as well as her inability to sway the county officials led to repeated negative votes by the county's legislators. Budgetary conditions were cited as one of the reasons for not funding a public health nurse, and Steffen's repeated efforts, although well-received by some in the community, were not viewed as reason for the county to spend its money on the services they received for free from the demonstration project that would be in effect for another year. Steffen left her position ahead of schedule in 1941, leaving the MCH demonstration position open until it was filled in January 1943 by another demonstration nurse, Hazel A. Nordley.

Apple described the differences that Nordley brought to the position. Whereas Steffen came from a large city, Nordley came from another more rural area in Wisconsin that perhaps made her more aware of those living in rural areas. Nordley's reports to the board reflected similar problems as Steffen's, but described the work with more detail and used a more positive tone when she wrote about the need, convincing the board of the need for public health nursing. In 1943 the Barron County board of legislators finally voted to support a position for a county nurse who would provide nursing services not just to children, but to all the families in the county. Apple (2011) wrote that there may have been several reasons for this change of heart (although she notes that the historical evidence is unclear or missing), including a change in the economy; the war effort, which depleted the county of physicians and nurses; the differences between the two demonstration nurses; and maybe "the board members had finally come to realize that modern medicine, particularly public health, offered much to the county" (p. 187). What is clear about the history of this particular story in Barron County is that nurses played a pivotal role in the implementation of public health initiatives and continue to do so today.

Using Apple's work to understand the kinds of decisions that needed to be made and should be made in relation to health care is important for us today. As nurse leaders make decisions about health care and how they can influence local and national legislators of the need for healthcare initiatives, historical studies such as the one completed by Apple offer perspective, context, and possible explanations for why and how decisions are made.

Other examples of historical research, such as the one published by Julie Fairman (2011), "The Visit: Nurse Practitioners and the Negotiation of Practice," examine the context in which the nurse practitioner establishes a relationship with patients and the space in which this relationship exists. Fairman's work builds on her larger study of the history of nurse practitioners and gives us insight into the many factors that influence the visit and what that means to the care provided. Fairman (2011) writes, "the clinical practice, then, is shaped by more than functional and technical tasks, but also by the partnership created through individual and personal interactions during the visit" (p. 189). The visit becomes even more complicated by other factors, including the "context of health care, the place of practice, and complexities of payment" (Fairman, 2011, p. 189). Negotiation between the physician and the nurse practitioner also impacts the visit and the relationships established during that visit with the patient. Fairman examines the visit in the context of the 1970s when early nurse practitioners were first establishing the relationships with physicians and both professions were struggling to maintain both professional authority and identity.

Another study by Helen Zuelzer (2011) examines pressure ulcers, a concern for healthcare providers that has lasted well over a century. Zuelzer studies the nursing interventions required to care for what were once called bedsores in, "'An Obstinate and Sometimes Gangrenous Sore': Prevention and Nursing Care of Bedsores, 1900 to 1940s." Zuelzer asks us to consider the new federal legislation that will hold acute care settings accountable if patients develop pressure ulcers, and traces the history of the kind of care that had been used and places it within the context of practice, lending perspective to the debate about the cause and care of this alteration in health. The chapter opens with the late actor Christopher Reeve's story about his traumatic injury after a fall off a horse and his struggles with living with a severe spinal cord injury. Zuelzer (2011) writes that when Reeve was interviewed he spoke about his care, his full-time staff, and the equipment to assist in his care, and that he was privileged to be able to afford this kind of care. Reeve also spoke about the many pressure ulcers he had, even with the extraordinary care he received. And even with this care, Zuelzer continued, Reeve died from an infection from a pressure ulcer.

Zuelzer examines the history of how nurses treated these bedsores, assessed them, and wrote about them in nursing texts, and they remain a persistent problem today. Zuelzer wrote, "descriptions of pressure injury, sites of injury and sources of injury pressure, friction, and shear, facilitated by moisture, remain remarkably unchanged" (p. 57). The debate about whether they can be avoided remains as well. Decisions nurses make today about interventions, such as care of pressure ulcers, have broad implications in terms of political, social, and economic factors. Historical evidence, hereto, offers us a better understanding of the kinds of care that nurses and other healthcare providers can offer and contributes to the leadership providing direction and making decisions about that care.

History as Evidence

Historical studies such as those facilitated by Keeling (2011), Connolly (2011), Apple (2011), Fairman (2011), and Zuelzer (2011) provide today's nurses with data of what was done in the past. They uncover the history of working nurses and make connections between then and now. Contemporary nurses struggle with decisions about advanced practice, nurse practice acts, federal legislation affecting Medicaid and Medicare reimbursement, epidemics, rural health care, and collaborating partnerships with physicians that would all benefit from the knowledge that these histories presented. Uncovering the history and analyzing its meaning contextualized by political, gender, ethnic, or racial factors informs not only the practice, but also the education and research and thus affects nursing outcomes today and in the future. Today's professionals can learn from the wisdom, knowledge, mistakes, and vision of those earlier nurses.

A number of years ago when I was an instructor in a community health course on the Lower East Side in New York City, one of the students, who was a registered nurse returning to school for a baccalaureate degree in nursing, was visiting a "client" of the Henry Street Settlement Home Health Care agency in the home. The student professionally worked as a cardiac care nurse and was proficient in providing high-level care using the latest technology in cardiac care. However, when she entered this client's home during the community clinical rotation, she said she was shocked at the odor emanating from the client's feet and had difficulty knowing what her responsibilities were in this case. She wanted to know what could be done for this client, because there were no medical orders and she felt she could not do anything without them.

The goal of the community experience at the Henry Street Settlement (where the visiting nursing service had separated from the agency in 1944) was to visit clients who received homemaking services in the home. Students were expected to develop a nursing plan of care after completing a nursing assessment of the client, reviewing the client's concerns and the homemaker's concerns, and completing an assessment of the home and community resources. When I visited the client's home with the student nurse and saw the caked-on dirt and smelled the odor from the feet, I asked the homemaker to prepare a basin of warm water so that we could soak the client's feet. We instituted a nursing intervention, bathing of the feet, so that we could further assess the skin color, the temperature, and the integrity of the skin. As we bathed the feet, the student spoke with the client and began to build trust with him and develop a rapport with the homemaker. Following the simple "nursing" procedure, the student patted the feet dry, continued to assess the feet, and began to teach the client about proper foot care.

The student said on the walk back to Henry Street that although she could operate efficiently in the hospital setting, the home-care setting created new challenges to her perceived role of the nurse. She was unaware of what visiting nurses did or had done in the past. She lacked historical perspective that might have assisted her in understanding this middle ground where nurses provide nursing care autonomously. The autonomous role that she was learning in the community clinical experience had ties with earlier nurses in the same community. Yet not knowing the past creates challenges for her and all nurses who make decisions in their practice.

History provides today's nurses with an "overarching conceptual framework that allows us to more fully understand the disparate meaning of nursing and the different experiences of nurses" (D'Antonio, 2003, p. 1). Lynaugh and Reverby (1987) said that history "provides us with the tools to examine the full range of human existence and to assess the constraints under which decisions are made" (p. 4). Without understanding nursing history, decisions are at risk of failing and repeating past errors. History provides a way of knowing and understanding what has gone on before, what is happening now, and what may be expected in the future. Fairman (2012) stated in a paper presented at the International Nursing History Conference, Nursing History in a Global Perspective that, "Modern nursing is a practice profession and a scientific discipline, and history is critical to its identity, cultural meaning, and relevance. . . . History provides meaning, and this meaning is infused into any area that we might want to study" (p. 8). If all knowledge has a historical dimension, then nurses need to take this dimension into account whenever a decision is made. All decisions, regardless of the decision-making approach that nurses may use, must include a historical dimension in the matrix. Like the case studies presented and the historical research identified, nurses can learn by understanding the past and using this understanding to support the kinds of decisions that they make today.

> History is alive, and the search for answers in history is useful for solving present difficulties, directing behavior, and accomplishing the objectives of the nursing profession. When the answers are found, it is not the end. It is the beginning (Austin, 1978, p. viii).

References

Apple, R. D. (2011). To avoid expense and suffering: Public health nurses and the struggle for health services. In P. D'Antonio & S. B. Lewenson (Eds.), *Nursing interventions through time: History as evidence* (pp. 173–188). New York: Springer Publishing Company.

Austin, A. L. (1978). Foreword. In M. Louise Fitzpatrick (Ed.), *Historical studies in nursing: Papers presented at the 15th annual Stewart Conference on Research in Nursing March 1977* (pp. vii–viii). New York: Teachers College Press.

Beck, M. B. (1934). Coordinating the teaching of sciences and nursing practice: Underlying scientific principles in nursing practice. *American Journal of Nursing, 34*(6), 579–586.

Christy, T. E. (1978). The hope of history. In M. L. Fitzpatrick (Ed.), *Historical studies in nursing: Papers presented at the 15th annual Stewart Conference on Research in Nursing March 1977* (pp. 3–11). New York: Teachers College Press.

Connolly, C. A. (2011). Determining children's "best interests" in the midst of an epidemic: A cautionary tale from history. In P. D'Antonio & S. B. Lewenson (Eds.), *Nursing interventions through time: History as evidence*. New York: Springer Publishing Company.

D'Antonio, P. (2003). Editor's note. *Nursing History Review, 11*, 1.

D'Antonio, P., & Fairman, J. (2010). Guest editorial: History matters. *Nursing Outlook, 58*, 113–114. doi: 10.1016/j.outlook.2010.01.004.

D'Antonio, P., & Lewenson, S. B. (Eds.) (2011). *Nursing interventions through time: History as evidence*. New York: Springer Publishing Company.

Fairman, J. A. (2008). Context and contingency in the history of post World War II nursing scholarship in the United States. *Journal of Nursing Scholarship, 40*(1), 4–11.

Fairman, J. A. (2012, August). *History counts: How nursing history shapes our understanding of health policy.* Draft of paper presented at the International Nursing History Conference, Nursing History in a Global Perspective, Kolding, Denmark.

Fairman, J. A. & D'Antonio, P. (2013). History counts: How history can shape our understanding of health policy. *Nursing Outlook, 61*(5), 346–352.

Fairman, J. A. (2011). The visit: Nurse practitioners and the negotiation of practice. In P. D'Antonio & S. B. Lewenson (Eds.), *Nursing interventions through time: History as evidence* (pp. 189–202). New York: Springer Publishing Company.

Harmer, B., & Henderson, V. (1940). *Textbook of the principles and practice of nursing* (4th ed., rev.). New York: MacMillan Company.

Keeling, A. W. (2001). Nursing history in the curriculum: Preparing nurses for the 21st century. AAHN position paper. Retrieved from http://aahn.org/position.html

Keeling, A. W. (2011). Treating influenza 1918 and 2010: Recycled interventions. In P. D'Antonio & S. B. Lewenson (Eds.), *Nursing interventions through time: History as evidence* (pp. 31–41). New York: Springer Publishing Company.

Keeling, A. W. & Lewenson, S. B. (2013). A nursing historical perspective on the medical home: Impact on health care policy. *Nursing Outlook, 61*(5), 360–366.

Lewenson, S. B. (1993). *Taking charge: Nursing, suffrage, and feminism in America, 1873–1920*. New York: Garland Publishing.

Lewenson, S. B. (2004). Integrating nursing history into the curriculum. *Journal of Professional Nursing, 20*(6), 347–380.

Lewenson, S. B. (2013). Historical research in nursing: A current outlook. In C. T. Beck (Ed.), *Routledge international handbook of qualitative nursing research* (pp. 256–267). London and New York: Routledge.

Lynaugh, J., & Reverby, S. (1987). Thoughts on the nature of history. *Nursing Research, 36*(1), 4, 69.

Madsen, W. (2008). Teaching history to nurses: Will this make me a better nurse? *Nurse Education Today, 28*, 524–529.

McManus, R. L. (1961). Nursing research—Its evolution. *American Journal of Nursing, 61*(4), 76–79. Retrieved from http://links.jstor.org/sici?sici=0002-936X%28196104%2961%3A4%3C76%3ANRIE%3E2.0.CO%3B2-P

Nelson, S., & Gordon, S. (2004). The rhetoric of rupture: Nursing as practice with a history? *Nursing Outlook, 52*, 255–261.

New York Board of Health (1897). *Annual report of the Board of Health of the Health Department of the City of New York for the year ending December 31, 1893*. New York: Martin B. Brown Company, Printers and Stationers.

New York Board of Health (1909). *Annual report of the Board of Health of the Department of Health of the City of New York VII, 1908*. New York: Martin B. Brown Company, Printers and Stationers.

Pape, T. M. (2003). Evidence-based nursing practice: To infinity and beyond. *Journal of Continuing Education in Nursing, 34*(4), 154–161.

Reiter, F. (1966). The nurse-clinician. *American Journal of Nursing, 66*(2), 272–280. Retrieved from http://www.jstor.org/stable/3419873

Roberts, M. (1939). Current events and trends in nursing. *American Journal of Nursing, 39*(1), 1–8. Retrieved from http://links.jstor.org/sici?sici=0002-936X%28193901%2939%3A1%3C1%3ACEATIN%3E2.0.CO%3B2-U

Strumpf, N. E., & Tomes, N. (1993). Restraining the troublesome patient: A historical perspective on a contemporary debate. *Nursing History Review*, 1, 1–24.

Toman, C., & Thifault, M.-C. (2012). Historical thinking and the shaping of nursing identity. *Nursing History Review*, 20, 184–204.

Wald, L. D. (1900). Work of women in municipal affairs. In *Proceedings of the Sixth Annual Convention of the American Society of Superintendents of Nurses* (pp. 54–57). Harrisburg, PA: Harrisburg Pub. Reprinted in Birnbach, N., & Lewenson, S. B. (Eds.) (1991). *First words: Selected addresses from the National League for Nursing, 1894–1933* (pp. 315–318). New York: National League for Nursing.

Wald, L. D. (1915). *The house on Henry Street*. New York: Henry Holt and Company.

Zuelzer, H. (2011). "An obstinate and sometimes gangrenous sore." In P. D'Antonio & S. B. Lewenson (Eds.), *Nursing interventions through time: History as evidence* (pp. 43–57). New York: Springer Publishing Company.

Chapter 3

Right or Wrong: Policy, Legal and Ethical Issues, and Decision-Making

Elizabeth Furlong

Nurses make decisions every day that must take into account health policy, laws, and ethical standards. Therefore, in order to make appropriate decisions, nurses require an understanding of how policy, laws, ethics, and nursing interface. This chapter provides a compelling case study that occurred in Nebraska and underscores the importance of nurses being constantly aware of proposed health policy, changing laws, petition drives, and ballot initiatives and their ethical implications. The Nebraska case study shows how proposed policy, legal issues, and ethical factors affect clinical nursing practice and how nurses must consider all aspects when making decisions in their practice.

Nebraska Case Study

In the summer and fall of 2006, a group of individuals from states outside of Nebraska wrote and financially funded a petition drive to obtain enough signatures to promote an amendment to the Nebraska state constitution (Stoddard, 2006a). The proposed amendment was titled "Nebraskans for a Humane Care Amendment." For the proponents, it would ensure a legal mandate that all individuals in Nebraska with a terminal condition would not have medical interventions, food, or water withheld or withdrawn. However, the amendment did include a statement that it would respect individuals' advance directives if they fully expressed a desire to withhold food and water in terminal conditions. The opponents of this petition had the following concerns:

- The initiative was from out of state.
- Only one or two Nebraskans had any involvement, which was a minimal legalistic engagement.
- If passed, the policy would create ethical dilemmas for patients, family members, and healthcare providers because the proposed amendment mandate did not reflect medical or ethical best practices for patients in terminal conditions.
- The amendment would take decision-making away from parents about their children's conditions.

In early September 2006, the Nebraska secretary of state ruled that the petition organizers had not obtained enough valid signatures to have the petition put on the November 2006 election ballot (Stoddard, 2006b). He disqualified many of the signatures that had been obtained for a variety of reasons; as a result, the amendment was not on the ballot for Nebraskans to decide in fall 2006. The policy activists, including many nurses, involved in resisting the 2006 policy were attentive in 2007 and 2008 in case another petition was initiated. In the 8 years since that proposed policy, there has not been another such policy initiation. Thus, although policy did not become a mandate for patients, family members, nurses, healthcare providers, institutions, and other policy and healthcare actors in the healthcare system, it is an exemplar case because of the intersection of policy, legal issues, and ethical aspects within the context of nursing practice.

Potential Implications for Practice

Had this amendment to the Nebraska state constitution been placed on the November 2006 ballot and voted on by Nebraskans, successfully passed, and become law, Nebraskan nurses would have had to follow the law or face penalties. Their nursing practice with patients in terminal conditions and their family members would have been mandated by this state constitutional amendment. A nurse who practices in a hospice setting, whether in a hospital, nursing home, or patient's home, would be mandated to continue administration of hydration and nutrition by artificial means even if not based on best practices.

In such a situation the nurse would be compelled to implement interventions because of the constitutional amendment (Nebraskans for Humane Care Committee, 2006). Thus, one can see the tension in decision-making between making decisions based on best practices, as in evidence-based practice, or decision-making based on proposed policy and law, but not based on clinical research.

Ethical concerns further complicate the nurse's decision-making process in this Nebraska case study. Nurses must balance their decisions based on what evidence-based practice dictates, what the law mandates, and what the ethical dilemma calls for. For example, perhaps the patient did not want the administration of hydration or nutrition but had not created an advance directive. Without that legal document, the patient, family, nurse, other healthcare providers, and others in the healthcare institution could not advocate for what the patient wants. Nurses have a responsibility to follow the American Nurses Association (ANA) Code of Ethics (American Nurses Association, 2012). In such a situation, nurses may well fail in their role and responsibility of being an advocate for the patient and to advocate for what the patient wants because they fear the penalty of law. Thus, nurses could be violating their own professional ethical code. They can, however, seek support when making their decisions (thereby perhaps decreasing their ethical dilemma) by considering the expectations of nurses in both the American Association of Colleges of Nursing (AACN) master's essentials and baccalaureate essentials documents. For example, in this Nebraska case study, nurse policy activists implemented all five of the knowledge outcomes found in the master's essentials; that is, (1) they analyzed the proposed policy for possible outcomes; (2) they participated in state policy activism; (3) they examined the policy and the legal effects of the proposed constitutional amendment for patients, family members, and nursing practice; (4) they based their activism on both research and the ANA Code of Ethics; and (5) they were strong advocates for patients, family members, the nursing profession, other healthcare providers, and the healthcare system (American Association of Colleges of Nursing, 2011).

What Nurses Need to Know and Do

The Nebraska case study signifies what nurses need to know and what nurses need to do to be in control of their profession and to be advocates for their patients. Nurses need to be able to read and understand legal language so they can analyze how that language will affect their practice and their patients. In this case, nurses needed to know the language of the Nebraska Humane Care Amendment, Section 30, which said (Nebraskans for Humane Care Committee, 2006):

> The fundamental human right to food and water should not be denied to any person, regardless of race, religion, ethnicity, nativity, disability, age, state of health, gender, or other characteristics: No entity with a legal duty of care for a person within its custody (including a hospital, orphanage, foster home, nursing home, sanitarium, skilled nursing facility, prison, jail, detainment center, corporation, business, institution or individual) may refuse, deny, or fail to provide food and water sustenance and nourishment, however delivered, to any such person if death or grave physical harm could reasonably result from such withholding and the person at risk can metabolize. Any such person so threatened with dehydration or starvation, any relative of such person, such person's legal guardian or surrogate, any public official with appropriate jurisdiction, or any protection and advocacy or ombudsman agency shall have legal standing to bring action for injunctive relief, damages and reasonable attorney's fees to uphold this standard of humane care. This section does not prohibit honoring the will of any person who, by means of a valid advance directive record, has fully expressly, and personally either authorized the withholding of food or water from himself or herself under specific conditions, or delegated that decision, under specific conditions, to one or more relatives or to another person unrelated to the entity with a legal duty of care.

It is important for nurses not only to be attentive to legal language and to understand that language, but also to critically think about how it affects their decisions. For example, a critique of the language in the proposed amendment reduced the patient to a biological determinant or to a biochemical definition of a human being, especially with the word *metabolize* (J. Welie, personal communication, October 23, 2006). Aside from the language being reductionistic of a human being, the choice of the word *metabolize* is incorrect because there is some metabolism after death. It is incongruent with the ethical practice of nurses to practice such reductionistic nursing care. Analysis of other language reflects that minors (and their families) would not have any decision-making rights. When nurses analyze potential laws that interfere with their ability to deliver quality ethical care to patients, they must intervene. Many nurses in Nebraska did exactly that by being part of the coalition group that formed in opposition to this proposed constitutional amendment.

Although most nurses think of laws when the word *legal* is evoked, the Nebraska case study educates nurses to another important dimension, which is a petition drive to add an amendment to a state constitution, the highest law of one's state. Further, no state law may be in contradiction to constitutional law. This petition drive was promoted by individuals and groups outside of Nebraska. A group, America at Its Best, with a postal address in Kalispell, Montana, was responsible for all of the $835,000 funding for the petition drive for the Nebraska Humane Care Amendment (Stoddard, 2006a). The same group provided almost all of the $861,998 for a second petition drive titled, Stop Over Spending Nebraska, whose purpose was to limit state spending. Only $1,998 was donated by people or entities others than the America at Its Best group (Stoddard, 2006a). This group listed the following national organizations as its supporters: Americans for Limited Government, Club for Growth, Funds for Democracy, and the National Taxpayers Union. In Nebraska, 113,721 valid signatures, or about 10 percent of registered voters, are needed on a petition ballot for it to be voted on at an election (Stoddard, 2006a, 2006b). The Nebraskans for Humane Care Committee turned in 137,200 signatures.

As noted earlier, nurses need to be able to analyze the use of language by others. Group titles and petition titles can be misleading and/or mean the exact opposite of what a citizen might think the language means. Many Nebraskans signed the petition thinking that the proposed amendment was a "good" thing because the title sounded positive (i.e., who could be against humane care?). Eventually, the Nebraska secretary of state found the group did not have enough valid signatures to put the petition on the ballot; about 20 percent of signatures had been declared invalid by county election officials (Stoddard, 2006b). Although this was because of a variety of reasons, one variable will be noted here—individuals who signed were given incorrect and/or fraudulent information when they were asked to sign the petition by the petition seekers. This has ramifications for nurses in their professional and civic lives. When nurses are aware of such misleading or fraudulent behavior on the part of amendment signature seekers, they must be activists. Such policy activity could take several forms: educating their colleagues, family, friends, and neighbors; writing letters to the editors of local newspapers; joining coalition groups engaged in the policy issue; and so forth.

Legal Aspects

Nurse Practice Act

One of the most important laws affecting nurses is the nurse practice act of their state because it provides the legal authority to practice their profession. The Nebraska case study emphasizes the importance of nurses being attentive to legal and ethical dimensions of their practice. This author believes every nurse has been educated and socialized to respect their nursing license. Nurses know about the necessity of passing the National Council Licensing Exam for Registered Nurses (NCLEX-RN), of obtaining and maintaining their nursing license, of knowing the nurse practice act in the state in which they are practicing nursing, of knowing and working within their nursing scope of practice, and of keeping informed about changes in nurse licensure issues. Further, because we live in a litigious society, nurses know the frequency of lawsuits and want to avoid possible loss of their license, termination of their employment, and involvement in a lawsuit as the defendant.

Thus, a core legal aspect for every nurse to know is the importance of her or his state nursing practice act. Because "nursing practice is regulated by each state through a board of nursing established by the state's government" (Wright & DeWitty, 2005, p. 3), nurses must understand what these laws are and how they dictate their practice. A nurse's professional life and economic livelihood are intimately related to the nurse practice act he or she needs to follow. Violating parts of that act can result in employment and licensure penalties. In every state a Board of Nursing has the responsibility and authority to: (1) issue nursing licenses, (2) regulate the practice of nursing, (3) enforce and interpret the specific state's nurse practice act, (4) promulgate administrative law (rules and regulations) that further clarifies the actual law, and (5) discipline nurses as necessary for the goal of ensuring the public's safety in the area of nursing care (Wright & DeWitty, 2005). In addition, a state Board of Nursing may give advisory opinions to nurses and other interested individuals with questions and concerns about the scope of nursing practice (Wright & DeWitty, 2005).

> Advisory opinions do not have the force or effect of law but generally are issued by a state board in response to evolving issues affecting nursing practice, such as mandatory overtime, or questions related to the scope of practice, such as the peripheral insertion of central venous catheter lines. (p. 4)

For example, in Nebraska there are 40 advisory opinions listed on the Nebraska State Board of Nursing Web site (Nebraska Health and Human Services, n.d.). Many of these opinions relate to the proposed amendment discussed in this chapter, including the topics of "Abandonment" and "Accountability for Professional Conduct of Nurses."

National Council of State Boards of Nursing

Web-based technology and use of the Multistate Nurse Licensure Compact for nurse licensure in many states have increased the helpfulness of the National Council of State Boards of Nursing (NCSBN) for nurses and nurse managers. The NCSBN provides a variety of services to the Boards of Nursing of all 50 states, the District of Columbia, and the five U.S. territories. These services include (Wright & DeWitty, 2005):

- Leadership on common concerns
- Development of the national nursing licensure examination (i.e., the NCLEX exam)
- Research and policy analysis
- Promulgation of national uniformity in the regulation of nursing practice

The technology system established by the NCSBN enables all state Boards of Nursing to have access to data regarding nurses' licenses and discipline information. Employees of any state Board of Nursing can enter or edit data, obtain data on past licensure or license discipline of nurses, and the like. Nursing employers can access this data for a fee. The general lay public cannot access this data. Besides verifying nurses' applicant license information, a Board of Nursing employee may also use the data system to review disciplinary information of a nurse and to electronically communicate between and among staff at other Boards of Nursing. This system is especially important given the increased mobility of many individuals and nurses in U.S. society, because of the Multistate Nurse Licensure Compact and the use of short-term travel nurses to meet patient needs. Nurses will find the Web site to be a helpful resource. If short-term travel nurses are coming and working in Nebraska, for example, they can use the Web pages of both the NCSBN and Nebraska's State Board of Nursing to better inform themselves of the kinds of laws, policies, and advisory opinions they must know to practice within their scope of practice in Nebraska.

The NCSBN took a leadership role in the 1990s when it studied and promoted a multistate Nurse Licensure Compact model for nursing licensure. This model has now been passed by state law in 24 states. See the NCSBN Web site for a listing and map of the states that have this model (www.ncsbn.org). This model, based on the driver's license model, allows a nurse to obtain a nursing license in their state of residency (home state) and then practice in other states that also belong to the Nurse Licensure Compact. The nurse is subject to the nurse practice act of the state in which the nurse is practicing. When practicing in multiple states that belong to the compact, the nurse has one nursing license: that of their home state (i.e., where the nurse resides). States have to pass laws to join the compact. This is yet another example of how laws and policy affect the practice of nursing.

It is the state Board of Nursing that addresses any complaints about a nurse; such complaints may begin the discipline process of that particular state board. Complaints about a nurse could come from a range of individuals: patients, family members, nursing or other work colleagues, employers, or individuals outside the work setting. "The most common complaints filed arise from known or suspected chemical impairment and abuse; drug diversion; criminal convictions; professional boundary violations; and practice deficiencies such as medication errors, documentation discrepancies or the failure to assess or intervene appropriately" (Wright & DeWitty, 2005, p. 6). Although particular practices may vary from one state Board of Nursing to another, there are three common steps for a nurse to anticipate after a discipline investigation has been initiated: the Board of Nursing will conduct an initial investigation, the nurse is informed, and then there will be further investigation, which results in a range of possible outcomes—from dismissal of the complaint to formal charges against the nurse. If a nurse is disciplined, the discipline action could be one of the following:

- An advisory letter
- A public reprimand
- Probation with monitoring by the Board of Nursing
- Suspension from nursing practice for a designated time period, which may include stipulations for reinstatement
- Revocation of one's nursing license, either permanently or nonpermanently

Because the discipline investigation context is adversarial and because one purpose of a state Board of Nursing is to protect the public regarding nursing care, nurses are advised to seek legal counsel with an experienced attorney in such an investigative situation.

A state constitution supersedes other state laws including a nurse practice act. If the Nebraska case study amendment had been voted on and passed by Nebraskans, nurses (and others) would have had to follow that constitutional amendment in terms of how they would treat all patients in the state. If the nurse chose not to (because of advocacy for the patient based on evidence-based nursing practice or ethical analysis), the nurse would be subject to penalty of law—and, further, would be in conflict with some goals of the nurse practice act administered by the Nebraska State Board of Nursing (to deliver competent, safe care to patients). Further, the nurse would be in conflict with her or his ANA Code of Ethics as well as other ethical principles.

It is beyond the purview of this chapter to include all aspects of the law and nursing. Nursing practice is affected by a multitude of federal, state, county, and city laws; by lawsuits against nurses; by rules and regulations; and by the precedent of court cases. In the following section, the Nebraskan case study is examined in terms of how policy and legal issues integrate with the ethical decision-making process.

Ethical Decision-Making

The Nebraska case study is also significant because of its ethical concerns. Nurses experience moral anguish when they engage in ethical dilemmas that concern patient care. Although there are many challenges facing nurses in the work environment (e.g., high patient-to-nurse ratios, mandatory overtime, worksite violence, and several others), it is the ethical and moral dilemmas that cause the most pain for nurses. The Nebraska case study is only one example of the kind of frustration, tension, and dilemmas that nurses have. Nurses experience moral anguish with the high patient-to-nurse ratio and knowing that best patient care is not being given. They experience moral anguish when mandated to work overtime—attempting to balance not abandoning their patients with their concern about not giving quality care and their fear of risking a lawsuit because of fatigue and increased risk of medical errors.

In making ethical decisions, three resources that are valuable for nurses are: (1) the ANA Code of Ethics, (2) an understanding of ethical principles, and (3) the AACN master's and baccalaureate essentials documents. The ANA Code of Ethics was revised in 2001. Although discussion of the Code in this part of the chapter concerns ethical dimensions, it also could have been emphasized in the previous policy and legal section of the chapter. For example, if a nurse is involved in a lawsuit, one of the factors that will be analyzed is: Did the nurse follow the ANA Code of Ethics? This is considered a standard of practice. If the nurse did not follow the Code of Ethics, the nurse's practice is considered substandard. Defense attorneys prepare and coach nurse defendants in lawsuits to be prepared for this line of questioning by the plaintiff's attorney (i.e., is the defendant nurse knowledgeable about and following the ANA Code of Ethics in her or his practice?).

Historically, one way of understanding ethics in the health system is to study ethics in terms of ethical principle—in other words, nonmaleficence, beneficence, fidelity, autonomy versus paternalism, veracity, and justice (Purtilo, 2005). This is the language commonly and routinely used and found in nursing and health literature, heard when participating in institutional ethics committees, and heard when other nurses and healthcare providers analyze ethical dilemmas. In addition to these, a discussion follows on the Ethics of Caring theory, which has emerged as another way of solving ethical dilemmas. This latter model comes from the work of Gilligan (1982), other feminists, and nurses.

The principle of *nonmaleficence* is not harming another (Purtilo, 2005). Nurses constantly aim to practice this ethical principle and hold it foremost in their practice. They do not want to harm patients;

further, they are healers, are ethical, and, given one aspect of this chapter, they do not want a lawsuit against them. In re-examining the Nebraskan case study, if there had been such a constitutional amendment in Nebraska, nurses would have had to choose between following the law and implementing what they know about risks and complications of sustained artificial hydration for dying patients. For example, there is clinical evidence that provision of hydration and nutrition in end-of-life illnesses may cause suffering and may increase aspiration pneumonia and bloating (Post & Whitehouse, 1995). Thus, a law could force nurses to harm a patient. There are a multitude of other examples that occur on a daily basis, where nurses make decisions, practice preventive interventions, revalidate orders, and use critical thinking and nursing judgment to prevent harm to patients. It can be said that the nurse is the patient's last defense. Nurses' attention to not causing harm to patients has greatly increased in the past decade because of the wide professional and lay media coverage of the problem of medical errors in the healthcare system (Milstead & Furlong, 2006).

The next principle is *beneficence*, which is bringing about good for the patient (Purtilo, 2005). In the Nebraskan case study, the proponents and the opponents of the proposed amendment differed on their analysis of this principle. The proponents saw this amendment as being positive for the patient. The opponents evaluated other dimensions to the issue (i.e., that it may bring clinical harm to some patients or that it violated other ethical principles, such as patient autonomy, fidelity, and justice). When reflecting on one's nursing practice, the usual situation is that every day a nurse works, she or he is making many decisions that are beneficent for the patient. To integrate with legal content discussed earlier in this chapter, the nurse practices beneficent nursing care that meets standards of care and the Code of Ethics. However, it should be easy for the reader to think of many situations for which there can be honest differences of opinion, values, and evaluation of situations—one person can evaluate that an intervention is harmful and another party can analyze the intervention as beneficent. This is the ethical dilemma and is the dilemma for this case study. There is a difference of analysis and evaluation of the beneficence of mandated hydration and nutrition for patients in terminal conditions. Three authors wrote articles during the summer of 2006 analyzing the Catholic moral tradition about end-of-life issues that apply to this case study. One writer, Shannon (2006) "sees the preservation of life at all costs as at least highly troubling, if not as a radical move against the Catholic medical ethics tradition" (p. 29). Drane (2006) analyzes the history of Catholic moral tradition and argues against the provision of artificial nutrition and hydration for all patients. Father Kevin O'Rourke (2006), a noted Catholic theologian and ethicist, argues for balancing costs with benefits when making decisions about artificial nutrition and hydration. He stresses the importance of decision-making by the patient, family members, and healthcare providers. His arguments for who should be the decision makers would be in opposition with the proposed amendment where the state government would be making the decision.

The third principle is *autonomy versus paternalism* (Purtilo, 2005). This means respecting the decision-making of the patient and/or the family members versus only considering the wishes of the healthcare providers in deciding treatment plans. There has been a paradigm shift in the United States during the past 50-plus years regarding this principle. Prior to about 1960, paternalism by healthcare providers (physicians) was the way decision-making was done. Physicians decided whether patients were told certain diagnoses and pressure was put on patients to always follow designated treatments (Friedlander, 1995). This model no longer receives the same emphasis; rather, the emphasis now centers on the autonomy of the patient, and, by extension, family members. There are many variables to explain this paradigm shift: (1) a U.S. population increasingly educated about their medical conditions, (2) a changed U.S. society where Americans no longer give deference or authority to several segments of society including the medical system, (3) a changed healthcare system for which interdisciplinary collaborativeness is recognized as the key to safe patient care versus dominance by physicians, and (4) Web technology with comprehensive easy access to medical and other knowledge.

Another current example of this ethical principle of autonomy being practiced can be seen in the federal Health Insurance Portability and Accountability Act (HIPAA). One could analyze that this particular federal law has emphasized and mandated one aspect of patient autonomy (i.e., that of patient decision-making in terms of who will have access to patient information).

This third principle of autonomy also applies to the Nebraskan case study. One could argue that the autonomy of patients was not being honored. However, it was not the traditional physician who was being paternalistic; rather, it was out-of-state organizers who were being paternalistic and deciding what was best medically for a population of Nebraska state residents. Had it passed, it then would have been the state government being paternalistic in end-of-life decisions. In retrospect, a partial evaluation of why the amendment did not elicit enough signatures in Nebraska integrates with this principle and with some other aspects of the culture of Nebraskans. In the United States generally, and in some states with a strong politically conservative ideology, such as Nebraska, there is an antigovernment philosophy (i.e., wanting the least amount of governmental intrusion in one's life). Having a state law mandating certain medical treatment would violate this Nebraskan philosophy. Another value held by Nebraskans is, if there is going to be government control, then the principle of subsidiarity should control (i.e., the government control should be as local as possible). It was definitely not perceived well by Nebraskans to have change agents from out-of-state fund and attempt to control state policy. At a state population level, Nebraskans do not like this kind of out-of-state influence and paternalism—whether it is regarding healthcare policy or other policy. Further, such out-of-state tactics are the antithesis of the singular populist history of this state. In addition to these issues, data from a 2007 survey conducted by the Nebraska Hospice & Palliative Care Organization described some of the wishes of Nebraskans relative to health care: 33 percent of Nebraskans had an advance directive, 96 percent "said it's important to be off machines that extend life, and 74 percent wouldn't want medical interventions to keep them alive as long as possible if they were dying" (Nebraska Hospice & Palliative Care Association "Survey Probes," 2007). Another data point related to this Nebraskan case study is that 75 percent of Nebraskans reported they felt that total physical dependency on others would be worse than death.

Besides the ethical consideration of autonomy versus paternalism, there is a legal counterpoint to the ethical dimension of this concept. A series of lawsuits originated from the classic 1914 lawsuit *Schloendorff v. New York Hospital*, which gave legal power and authority to the individual regarding what happens to his or her body (*autonomy*) (Menikoff, 2001). Some of these lawsuits also related to the necessity of having informed consent between a healthcare provider and a patient. This third principle of autonomy versus paternalism is deeply rooted in both ethics and the law in this country. The proposed constitutional amendment would have contradicted the history of both ethics and law in this regard.

Nurses in the early twenty-first century recognize the autonomy of patients and family members. If the proposed amendment of the Nebraskan case study had been enacted into law, how would a Nebraska nurse work within this ethical dilemma? Suppose the nurse practices in a hospice setting, the patient has no "fully expressed" advance directive, but the family knows (from many conversations with the dying patient) that he did not want prolonged artificial hydration. What does the nurse do? Follow the law and implement the mandated policy? What about the nurse's responsibility to follow the ethical principle of respecting the patient's autonomy? What about the nurse's responsibility to follow the ANA's Code of Ethics and advocate for patients? What about the nurse's responsibility to follow best practices?

Another ethical principle is that of *justice* (Purtilo, 2005), which relates to the nurse's position (professionally and personally) whereby the nurse has the ability to distribute benefits and burdens to individuals and to society. A beginning way to think about the justice imperative is to reflect on and evaluate one day in a clinical setting as a nurse. How did I spend my time? If I was assigned several patients, how did I spend my time? Did I spend it justly? What would be the several patients' perspectives, if questioned, of how I divided my time among them? How would I justify my time with each of them? The reader can think of many more justice issues in nursing. For example, is it just (to patients and to oneself) to continue working on a unit where there is persistent understaffing? Is it just (to patients and to oneself) to continue working in an environment where there is consistent mandatory overtime? Also, there are broader issues in the healthcare system, such as how total healthcare resources should be allocated.

There could be many ways to apply this Nebraskan case study to the ethical principle of justice, but just two will be given here. Individuals' behaviors are influenced by many laws and regulations: federal, state, county, and city. The United States—its Constitution and its laws—was forged on a balance between federal and state laws. There is a strong history of Americans wanting any law or regulation to be at the most local level versus a federal law (i.e., the concept of *subsidiarity*). Is it just for individuals outside of one state to make policy for people residing in another state? Is it just to use language—"Nebraskans for a Humane Care Amendment"—when some individuals would analyze the language as not being totally truthful? Another area of justice relates to cost. Healthcare costs have always been a significant driver of reform in the system and have affected whether many individuals seek or receive health care. Is it just, from a cost perspective, to mandate sustained hydration and nutrition for all?

In addition to analyzing ethical dilemmas based on these four principles, another model to use is the Ethics of Caring. This model of analysis builds on the work of Carol Gilligan (1982) who expanded on Lawrence Kohlberg's model of moral development of individuals, which was at the time the dominant theory for understanding this aspect of individuals. However, Gilligan, one of his graduate students, continued his research—but with girls. She noted differences in how girls, boys, women, and men conceptualized ethical dilemmas (Beauchamp & Childress, 2001; Brannigan & Boss, 2001; Purtilo, 2005). This model of ethical analysis emphasizes relationships, caring for others, listening to others' stories, and balancing justice issues with compassion. Although there is not a strict gender division, women tend to embrace a conception of considering the total context of a situation, maintaining and nurturing relationships, and being caring when considering an ethical dilemma. Men tend to evaluate ethical dilemmas more in justice terminology and with more impartial, dispassionate conflict resolution.

Because of the dominance of women in the nursing profession, the Ethic of Care is further emphasized, not only because of the numerical strength of women nurses, but also because a core essence of nursing is caring. Healthcare providers and the lay public usually associate caring with nurses and curing with physicians. In the past 25 years, many nurses have written about Gilligan's work and applied it to nursing. An important aspect of the Ethic of Caring is narrative ethics requiring "that all voices be considered before the situation is assessed for its moral significance" (Purtilo, 2005, p. 56). In the Nebraskan case study, had all voices been heard?

Nebraska Nurses Respond to the Nebraska Amendment

Nebraska nurses, in their roles as leaders, responded to the proposed petition drive that did not get on the ballot in November 2006, using the media to transmit their concerns, individual lobbying, and so forth. Amy Haddad (2006), director of the Center for Health Policy and Ethics (CHPE) at Creighton University and a nurse, wrote an editorial for the *Omaha World Herald* discussing the issue and raising concerns. For many individuals, this was the first time that concerns with the petition drive were in the public media. Because of the controversy surrounding the issue, Haddad first shared her writing with all levels of university administrators and legal counsel. Second, the Center for Health Policy and Ethics hosted a brown-bag lunch meeting on the issues the amendment raised. Invited speakers included a theology professor, an attorney, and an ethicist from the CHPE who is educated as a physician and attorney as well as an ethicist. Third, the CHPE developed a summary position statement and distributed that statement to attendees. The statement emphasized four areas of concern:

1. Decision-making would be taken from family members and given to the state unless there was a living will with specific language or an appropriate power of attorney.
2. A competent patient could not refuse treatment nor grant or withhold informed consent.
3. The amendment required a procedure that may not help a patient; rather it might cause discomfort and/or hasten death.
4. The amendment proponents presented no evidence of a current concern or problem with patients in Nebraska.

Proponents were presuming that only the use of law and potential legal punishment would assure best care at the end of life. A large group of concerned healthcare providers, other individuals, and healthcare agencies formed a coalition to address the concerns they had with this proposed amendment. This group held many meetings, planned strategies, and educated the public. It recognized that the amendment, although not on the ballot in the fall of 2006 because of technical reasons, might be an issue again in fall 2008. One example of the kind of education and analysis the group provided was a lengthy side-by-side column analysis of current law and practice in Nebraska with provisions of the proposed amendment (R. Anderson, personal communication, September 2006). Analysis by attorney Anderson and others noted the poor legal construction of the proposed amendment because many phrases were vague, language was not defined, and many phrases were open to interpretation. Another kind of education and analysis was presented by the many nurses who participated in this coalition and who shared their clinical, theoretical, and research knowledge. Many of these nurses were hospice nurses, and their knowledge of both dying patients and the literature greatly contributed to others' understanding. In an earlier section of this chapter, it was noted that the petition group, America at Its Best, spent $835,000 on education and lobbying of voters to get on the ballot. Education of healthcare professionals, patients, families, and voters was done on a shoestring budget by the nurses and others. As noted earlier in this chapter, the petition was not reinitiated in 2008.

Reaction to the "Out-of-State" Initiative

During spring 2007, several Nebraska state senators introduced three state laws to address concerns raised by the proposed 2006 constitutional amendment discussed in this chapter. First, Senator Ray Aguilar introduced Legislative Bill 311, which was unanimously voted out of the Government, Military and Veterans Affairs Committee (Nebraska Legislature, 2007). This bill would change provisions relating to petition signature verification and have such provisions conform to the court case of *Stenberg v. Moore*. The second bill, introduced by Senator Bill Avery, would change signature thresholds for both constitutional amendments and statutory initiatives (Nebraska Legislature, 2007). His proposed bill, which moved forward from the same unicameral legislative committee by a vote of 6–1, would increase the required number of signatures on constitutional amendments from 10 percent of the state's registered voters to 15 percent. His intent was to make it more difficult to change the state constitution. His and other senators' concerns were the issues discussed in this case study and other petition drives in Nebraska since 1990. Senator Avery said, "I also have deep respect for our state constitution. It deserves to be protected from the desires and whims of out-of-state organizations. It's not written in pencil so that whoever has the biggest eraser can come in and erase it all willy-nilly" (Nebraska Legislature, 2007, p. 7). The third bill, introduced by Senator DiAnna Schimek, passed the first of three necessary rounds of voting in the full unicameral session by a 31–11 vote on February 1, 2007 (Reed, 2007). This bill would prohibit petition circulators from being paid per signature when they are employed for such work. Again, the origin of this bill related to the concerns and frustrations state senators and others had with the issues discussed in the Nebraska case study. Sen. John Harms's argument during the unicameral discussion was reflective of many senators: "That's what got people fired off, it was people coming here from out of state, with no idea about the issues in Nebraska. . . . It was millionaires putting money into telling Nebraskans what to do. That's wrong" (Reed, 2007, p. B2). The two bills introduced by Senators Aguilar and Schimek were passed on March 7th, 2007 and February 19th, 2008; the bill introduced by Senator Avery was indefinitely postponed on April 17, 2008. In summary, the introduction of these three state laws (with one relying on the judicial outcomes of a court case) demonstrated other important ways that legal decisions affect nursing in addition to constitutional amendments (initiation of state laws and court cases). Nurses in Nebraska were active in lobbying measures on these bills.

In the years since the stoppage of this petition, other policy activism has been occurring in Nebraska on this topic. This advocacy, titled "It's All About the Conversation," is the beginning effort of a large multidisciplinary task force of, again, interested policy activists on the issues of end-of-life care and advance care planning. However, since its beginning in April 2012, the policy dynamics have been far different than what was seen in the 2006 case study. This group was started within Nebraska, by Nebraskans, and is a group that is multidisciplinary, inclusive, and intentionally representative of any who have interests in and concerns for these aspects of the healthcare system. Some examples of policy actors are chaplains; community members; emergency medical services employees; nurses; physicians; representatives of nursing homes, long-term care settings, and hospices; and state government health and human services employees. This group met in November 2012 to forge its mission statement. It is incorporating the results of three research studies done by the Nebraska Hospice & Palliative Care Association, yet another indicator of the concern for what the population of this one Midwestern state wants for their health care at the end of life. Of special import to this chapter is that one important leadership individual in the group is an advance practice nurse implementing a policy role that the essentials document calls for. Although the three survey studies are one indicator of ongoing interest in this aspect of the healthcare system, another indicator is the frequent use of the Physician Orders for Life-Sustaining Treatment (POLST) directives by physicians in three mid-state towns of Columbus, Kearney, and Norfolk. (H. Chapple, personal communication, November 6, 2012). The latter will be one model of end-of-life care the group will discuss. Thus, when comparing the two case studies (2006 and 2012), one of a government petition policy and one of a private sector policy, one can analyze very different traits regarding each proposed policy approach. Further, one can affirm the activism and health policy competencies of nurses in each case study to promote population health status.

Nurses must be cognizant of the many influences that affect decision-making and nurses' practice on a daily basis. This text gives the nurse insight into others' decision-making including patients, family members, healthcare providers, institutional administrators, and policy advocates. Although this chapter has focused on some policy, legal, and ethical content, the 2006 Nebraska case study demonstrated why and how easily one's clinical nursing practice can be significantly altered because of proposed policy and legal activities that may cause nurses legal, ethical, and professional difficulties. Rentmeester (2006) stated:

> In negotiating uncertainties and responding to interesting, important, and complex questions and dilemmas in healthcare, it appears that healthcare professionals cannot rely solely on legal experts. Rather, they must carefully discern and collegially discuss moral reasons to respond with care to patients and to one another in difficult cases. (p. 32)

The Nebraska case study exemplifies one complex dilemma in patient care: policy, law, ethics, and nurses. They interact with each other in dramatic ways. Nurses, as leaders, need to be prepared for these challenges.

References

American Association of Colleges of Nursing (2011). *The essentials of master's education in nursing*. Retrieved from http://www.aacn.nche.edu/education-resources/masters-essentials-resource-center

American Nurses Association (2012). *Code of ethics*. Retrieved from http://www.nursingworld.org/codeofethics

Beauchamp, T. L., & Childress, J. F. (2001). *Principles of biomedical ethics*. New York: Oxford University Press.

Brannigan, M. C., & Boss, J. A. (2001). *Healthcare ethics in a diverse society*. Mountain View, CA: Mayfield Publishing Company.

Drane, J. F. (2006). Stopping nutrition and hydration technologies: A conflict between traditional Catholic ethics and church authority. *Christian Bioethics, 12*, 11–28.

Friedlander, W. J. (1995). The evolution of informed consent in American medicine. *Perspectives in Biology and Medicine, 38*(3), 498–510.

Gilligan, C. (1982). *In a different voice: Psychological theory and women's development.* Cambridge, MA: Harvard University Press.

Haddad, A. (2006, July 4). Midlands voices: Health care change would be inhumane. *Omaha World Herald*, Editorial/Opinion page. Retrieved from http://chpte.creighton.edu/publications/focusfall-2006/story_directors.htm

Menikoff, J. (2001). *Law and bioethics.* Washington, DC: Georgetown Press.

Milstead, J. A., & Furlong, E. (2006). *Handbook of nursing leadership: Creative skills for a culture of safety*. Sudbury, MA: Jones & Bartlett.

Nebraska Health and Human Services (n.d.). *Advisory opinions.* Retrieved from http://www.hhs.state.ne.us/crl/nursing/Rn-Lpn/advisory.htm

Nebraska Hospice & Palliative Care Association (2007, February 5). Survey probes attitudes on death, dying. *Omaha World Herald*, p. E1.

Nebraskans for Humane Care Committee (2006). *Nebraskans for Humane Care.* Retrieved from http://www.nehumanecare.com

Nebraska Legislature, Government, Military & Veterans Affairs Committee (2007). Bills would change petition requirements. *Unicameral Update, XXX*(4), 1, 7.

O'Rourke, K. (2006). Reflections on the papal allocution concerning care for persistent vegetative state patients. *Christian Bioethics, 12*, 83–97.

Post, S., & Whitehouse, P. (1995). Fairhill guidelines on ethics of the care of people with Alzheimer's disease: A clinical summary. *Journal of the American Geriatrics Society, 43*, 1423–1429.

Purtilo, R. (2005). *Ethical dimensions in the health professions* (4th ed.). Philadelphia: Elsevier Saunders.

Reed, L. (2007, February 2). Petition restrictions advance. *Omaha World Herald*, pp. B1–2.

Rentmeester, C. A. (2006). What's legal? What's moral? What's the difference? A guide for teaching residents. *American Journal of Bioethics, 6*(4), 31–32.

Shannon, T. A. (2006). Nutrition and hydration: An analysis of the recent papal statement in the light of the Roman Catholic bioethical tradition. *Christian Bioethics, 12*, 29–41.

Stoddard, M. (2006a, August 10). Outsiders fueled two petition drives. *Omaha World Herald*, pp. B1–2.

Stoddard, M. (2006b, September 19). Humane care vote could be in '08. *Omaha World Herald*, p. A1.

Wright, L. D., & DeWitty, V .P. (2005). *Legal basics for professional nursing practice.* Silver Springs, MD: Center for American Nurses.

Chapter 4

More than Prayer: Spirituality and Decision-Making

Joy Buck

"I let go of him once, I do not think that I can bear to do it again." That is what Martha said to the ICU nurse after the surgeon told her that her husband of 2 years was critically ill. Martha and Hal, both 55, quickly fell in love after meeting at a church function and married a year later. Both felt blessed that they had finally found their soul mate. On their first anniversary, they learned that Hal had a mass in his right lung. After surgery to remove the lung, they learned that it was serious and he had stage four lung cancer. He and his wife prayed over the situation and decided not to have chemotherapy that would ultimately only prolong his life rather than cure the cancer. The oncologist disagreed but Hal and Martha were strong in their faith and resolute. Ultimately, he supported them in their decision.

Hal did well for 6 months. He and Martha traveled extensively and enjoyed life to the fullest. Then Hal got sick and was hospitalized with a necrotizing pneumonia that was not responding to treatment. The nurses on the floor were drawn to the couple and touched by their love and courage. The nurses were mixed, however, about the do not resuscitate (DNR) order on his chart. When Hal got into respiratory distress, Martha was at his bedside. The charge nurse called the pulmonologist who responded just as Hal went into respiratory arrest. They initiated cardiopulmonary resuscitation (CPR), and he was intubated and resuscitated despite the DNR order. Martha was in a state of panic when the pulmonologist spoke to her about his actions. His rationale was that they could treat the pneumonia best by placing Hal on a ventilator and transferring him to the ICU where the nurses could monitor him carefully.

Martha agreed to this course of action and was relieved when Hal initially responded to treatment. He was awake, tolerated the ventilator well, and communicated effectively through nonverbal gestures and by writing notes. Pat, an ICU nurse, shared the couples' religious faith and prayed with them daily for his healing. Kathy, another ICU nurse, took care of him on the weekends. Kathy spent a lot of time listening to them as they spoke about their deep love, faith, and gratefulness that they had the time they had together. There was something about Kathy that was intangible, but both Hal and Martha knew that they could trust her.

Kathy was not particularly religious but she had firm ethical values and beliefs regarding the right to self-determination and her role as an advocate. She had a particular interest in palliative care and integrating its concepts into care of the seriously and critically ill. In the absence of a palliative care team in the hospital, she often facilitated conversations among patients and families about their care preferences and goal clarification associated with treatment options, prognosis, and quality of life. At times she intervened with physicians on behalf of the patient or family member. In some cases, she opened the door to communication with the physician resulting in a better alignment of medical treatment with the patient and family goals and preferences. In this case, the pulmonologist had one goal in mind—to cure the pneumonia. He had strong religious convictions about the sanctity of life and professional obligation to cure disease.

The second weekend Kathy took care of Hal, he required higher ventilator settings. Martha was a constant at Hal's bedside, often holding his hand and sharing stories about precious times that they had together. Although Hal was still engaged, he seemed to be distancing himself and was somewhat pensive. On Sunday evening after Martha left, Kathy asked him how he was doing and how she could help. He knew that he was getting worse and wrote, "Help her—when she is ready." She documented it on the chart and spoke to the other ICU nurses about what he had written.

On Hal's third weekend in the ICU, Kathy noted a marked difference in his condition. He was septic and the pulmonologist ordered aggressive measures to combat it; a surgeon was called to insert another central line. The surgeon explained to Martha how poor Hal's prognosis was and asked if she wanted them to continue with aggressive treatment. Kathy waited with Martha when he left and asked what she wanted to do and how she could help. When she returned to the ICU, Hal had a cardiac arrest and the pulmonologist insisted on resuscitation. Kathy could not participate in the code—she knew that it was contrary to Hal's wishes. A colleague took her place as she sat and prayed with Martha. When the surgeon came to tell them that Hal had died, she held Martha as she cried. On Monday morning, Kathy referred the case to the ethics committee for a review and tendered her resignation to the ICU nurse manager. She loved the ICU and had tried her best to improve the care of critically ill patients and their families, but she could no longer participate in medical management of patients that she believed was morally reprehensible.

Kathy's story is just one example of the moral distress that nurses experience when facing situations in the clinical setting. This scenario reflects the extent to which diverse religious and spiritual beliefs shape personal and clinical decision-making in distinct ways. In this case, a physician recommended a specific course of action that was inconsistent with Hal's expressed wishes and DNR order. He did so because of his religious convictions and what he considered his professional obligation to preserve life. Martha was in crisis. In the moment, she believed the pulmonologist when he said that he could cure Hal of the pneumonia—a glimmer of hope in the face of devastating loss. Pat, who supported Martha's decision and the pulmonologist's actions, prayed with them for a miracle. She deeply believed that life should be preserved—ultimately it was in God's hands but they needed to use the medical technology and tools they had to keep Hal alive. Kathy also supported the couple through what was, in her mind, an untenable situation. She had deeply held cultural values, and from her perspective, the pulmonologist had acted against Hal's and Martha's best interests and preferences. In doing so, he caused unnecessary physical, emotional, and psychological harm that left Martha with over $100,000 in medical bills in addition to funeral costs.

Nurses are often confronted with difficult decisions about how to respond in different clinical situations. This is particularly true when caring for persons with serious illness. If you had been involved with Hal's care, what would you have done? How would you have reconciled your personal values, religious convictions, professional ethics, and obligations, given the situation?

Spirituality and Decision-Making Defined

Historically, faith traditions have played a dominant role in the development of the nursing profession (O'Brien, 1999; Shelley & Miller, 1999). Today, there is consensus that greater attention should be given to the spiritual dimensions of nursing care, but there is no clear direction about what spiritual care is or under what circumstances it is appropriate or desirable. The term *spirituality* means different things to different people. The literature suggests that classifications of spirituality range from the strictly religious to the strictly secular (van Leeuwen, Tiesinga, Post, & Jochemsen, 2006). In the case study, the pulmonologist and Pat made treatment and care decisions based on a religious doctrine that values life at all costs. This is consistent with the traditional definition of spirituality as ". . . something that in ecclesiastical law belongs to the church or to a cleric" (Merriam-Webster, 2003). Kathy, by contrast, acted in a manner consistent with her interpretation of spirituality as a quest for meaning not associated with religious beliefs, rituals, or practices. Rather, it was grounded in her deep belief in care that is respectful of the human condition, the nature of loss, and Hal and Martha's desire for quality of life and a peaceful death.

Although no common definition of spirituality exists, it has been defined as relating to the nature of the spirit, being intangible or nonmaterial, and concerning or affecting the soul (American Heritage, 1992). Nurse authors and theorists have explored the meaning of spirituality in nursing practice (Buck, 2007; Humphreys, 2001; McSherry & Cash, 2004; Post-White et al., 1996; Tanyi, 2002). When combined, definitions of spirituality in nursing include the elements of transcendence, mystery, connectedness, meaning and purpose, hope, higher power, and relationships (Tanyi, 2002; van Leeuwen et al., 2006). Some researchers have found Antonovsky's Salutogenic Model of Health (1979) with its central construct, sense of coherence, useful. This model posits that sense of coherence is essential to wellness or the source of health. *Sense of coherence* is defined as

> ...a global orientation that expresses the extent to which one has a pervasive, enduring though dynamic feeling of confidence that (1) the stimuli deriving from one's internal and external environments in the course of living are structured, predictable and explicable; (2) the resources are available to one to meet the demands posed by these stimuli; and (3) these demands are challenges, worthy of investment and engagement. (Antonovsky, 1987, p. 19)

Sense of coherence is conceptually similar to hope and has three key components (Antonovsky, 1979, 1987):

1. *Comprehensibility:* A belief that things happen in an orderly and predictable fashion and a sense that you can understand events in your life and reasonably predict what will happen in the future
2. *Manageability:* A belief that you have the skills or ability, the support, the help, or the resources necessary to take care of things, and that things are manageable and within your control
3. *Meaningfulness:* A belief that things in life are interesting and a source of satisfaction, that things are really worth it, and that there is good reason or purpose to care about what happens

Of these three components, Antonovsky believed that *meaningfulness* was the most important because if a person has no meaning, there is no motivation to comprehend and manage life's challenges and stress.

In a study of hopefulness in cancer patients, the authors identified five central themes that increased sense of coherence and quality of life in participants, including finding meaning and having affirming relationships (Post-White et al., 1996). McSherry and Cash (2004) proposed a taxonomy of spirituality that included the following descriptors: theistic, or a belief in a supreme being or deity; religious, a belief in God and certain religious practices, rituals, and customs; language, including expressions of inner peace and strength; social, political, and cultural ideologies; phenomenological, the process of learning through experiences; existential, a semantic philosophy of life and being; quality of life; and mystical, the relationship among the transcendent, interpersonal, and transpersonal.

For the purposes of this chapter, we provide a broad definition of spirituality: a personal search for meaning that may or may not be related to religion and that is used as a basis to explore the relevance of spiritual beliefs in end-of-life decision-making from the perspective of nurses, patients, and families. The term *religious* is used for specific religious practices, orthodoxy, and values.

Beginning with an examination of the historical relevance of spirituality to nursing care, this chapter uses a series of case studies to investigate how spiritual and religious beliefs shape individual perceptions, interpretations, and interactions among and between health professionals, patients, and their families. The chapter concludes with recommendations and resources to assist nurses to understand their own spirituality and values while appreciating those of their patients, families, and communities.

Rites and Rights of Living and Dying

Until the middle of the twentieth century, care for the dying was firmly within the domain of home, family, and religion (Buck, 2007, 2010; Buhler-Wilkerson, 2001; Smith & Nickel, 1999). Family members, primarily women, cared for the dying person and prepared the body for burial when they died. For those with financial means, private nurses were hired to provide care. The terminally ill without family or financial means to pay for care in voluntary hospitals were sent to almshouses or asylums until they died—or in some circumstances they were cared for in specialized homes for the dying. Many of these homes, though not all, were founded by groups of the Christian or Jewish faith. These groups varied in their approaches to management of the death bed and rituals prior to and after death—yet, they were bound by a commitment to religious ideals and beliefs that called them to serve the most vulnerable in their midst (Buck, 2007; Clark, 1997; Humphreys, 2001; Siebold, 1992; Walsh, 1929).

By the late 1940s, a series of social, political, and economic forces resulted in the transition of care for the dying from home to hospital. This move had a profound impact on the process of dying and the important role of family and religion within that process. As the locus of care and control over death changed from person and family to medical professionals, the context of the dying moved from the moral order to the technical order. Cassel (1974) characterized death in the moral order as a process that allowed for "caring for" and rituals to ease the passage of the mortal body to the immortal soul. In contrast, death in the technical order was a definitive event marked by cessation of certain biological functions, such as breathing or a beating heart. The focus of medical care was not the person or spirit, but rather the science and technology of organ function measurement. Dying in the technical order reduced death to a series of events and changes in biological function and indicated the end of life. The emergence of organ transplantation and medical technology to measure brain waves resulted in a change of the definition of death from the heart and lungs to the brain to allow for the harvesting of "live" organs from brain-dead individuals. Whereas at one time death was considered a natural occurrence, its medicalization transformed it into a distinctly unnatural event.

During the 1960s, research funded by the U.S. Public Health Service Division of Nursing documented the stark realities of institutionalized dying: Pain control was virtually nonexistent and terminally ill cancer patients frequently died in a room at the end of the hall, in exquisite pain and alone (Duff & Hollingshead, 1968; Glaser & Strauss, 1965, 1968; Quint, 1967; Sudnow, 1967). Social movements outside the walls of medical institutions began to clamor for the reform of care provided within. The civil and women's rights, death with dignity, and consumer movements laid a foundation for a growing public discourse about the quality of life, patients' rights, and the place of informed consent in the medical system. Stories of how cancer patients suffered while undergoing aggressive curative treatment were widely publicized in the popular press. Despite the promise of curative medicine, many began to wonder if the quest for cure was worth the human toll in suffering (Buck, 2007).

Although there were many people involved with the death and dying movements that emerged during the twentieth century, it was U.S. psychiatrist Elisabeth Kübler-Ross who played a pivotal role in stimulating serious reforms. She helped revolutionize society's conceptualization of death, dying, and bereavement with the publication of her book, *On Death and Dying*, in 1969. Despite her critics, and there were many, Kübler-Ross's writings reached international lay and professional audiences. In the early 1970s, nurses commonly cited Kübler-Ross as having the greatest influence on their attitudes toward death. Journalists attributed Kübler-Ross as single-handedly turning around an entire generation of opinion makers on the topic (Filene, 1998).

In the mid-1970s, media coverage of the Karen Ann Quinlan case further propelled the "right-to-die movement" into the collective U.S. consciousness and the movement from incipiency into coalescence. The landmark Quinlan case revolved around a family's wish to withdraw life-sustaining medical intervention, specifically a ventilator, from Karen Ann because she was deemed to be in a persistent, vegetative state. The decision in this case was not based on her brain or organ death, or extreme suffering, but rather on the basis of the quality of her life. Was living in a persistent vegetative state a life that should be sustained? Public debate on this issue was centered on questions about an individual's right to self-determination, the rights of surrogates acting on behalf of others, determinations of the quality and futility of life, the conditions under which one might choose to end life, and protections for those who helped them die in the manner they chose—all issues we continue to debate today (Buck, 2005; Filene, 1998; Webb, 1997).

It was within this context that the hospice movement emerged. Florence Wald, the acknowledged "nurse midwife" of the hospice movement in the United States, was dean of the Yale School of Nursing when she first heard British physician Cicely Saunders speak about hospice in 1963. A self-identified idealist, Wald was drawn to the hospice concept and the centrality of nursing within it. Hospice resonated to the core of her being and she made a commitment to transplant Saunders's vision of hospice onto U.S. soil (Buck, 2004; Krisman-Scott, 2001). Unlike Cicely Saunders, who cited her evangelistic Christian faith as being foundational to her commitment to the care of the terminally ill, Wald was motivated by a deep sense of moral obligation to humanity and social justice (Buck, 2011; Clark, 1998; du Boulay, 1984). She found a strong ally in Reverend Edward Dobihal, an evangelistic Methodist minister with a background in pastoral counseling and bereavement. Together, they initiated a multidisciplinary effort to research and reform care for the dying. In 1971, they, along with a growing group of supporters, founded a nonprofit organization, Hospice, Inc. By 1974, the group had funding to open the first modern hospice home care program, and hospice was well on its way to becoming a national phenomenon and a reimbursable model of care under the Medicare program (Buck, 2004, 2011).

This brief historical overview provides insights into the significance of religious and secular ideals to twentieth-century terminal care reform efforts. The religious call to care for the dying is most explicitly demonstrated with the evolution of religious homes for the dying in the United States, some of which are still operational (Buck, 2006). As hospice struck a responsive chord in the United States, research revealed that when compared to nurses in standard settings, hospice nurses were characterized as having deep spiritual faith and a well-developed commitment to finding meaning in life through service to others (Amenta, 1984; Pannier, 1980). Many of the early hospice training programs for staff and volunteers focused on the highly philosophical notions of the meaning of life and death, "being with," and ministering to and caring for dying patients and their families. These groups faced challenges in determining what spiritual care meant in a religiously plural society—yet, these discussions led to the reintroduction of spirituality as an explicit and essential component of care for the terminally ill (Buck, 2007).

The U.S. hospice and subsequent palliative care movements cut across many societal boundaries and reframed discussions about the appropriate care for persons with life-limiting and serious illness. Yet, many significant challenges remain in our current models of hospice and palliative care. As medical and technological advances provide more treatment options, societal debates over the moral implications of treatment withdrawal have become increasingly contentious and polarized. Nurses are often involved with the care of individuals and families in crisis (Weigand & Funk, 2012). As such, it is important that they reflect on their own spirituality and how their beliefs shape interactions with their colleagues and patients and their families who are entrusted to their care.

Spirituality and Decision-Making in Contemporary Times

Although it is clear that deeply held spiritual beliefs shaped career and end-of-life care decisions in the past, in what ways do they shape these issues today? Spiritual faith has been shown to be a protective factor during times of transition and crisis. The terms *spirituality* and *religion* are often used interchangeably and seen as being protective concepts (Sessanna, Finnell, Underhill, & Peng, 2011). It is important to note, however, that the concept of religiosity, or the quality of being religious and at times excessive devotion to religion, is not necessarily synonymous with having faith or being spiritual. In some circumstances, religiosity has been associated with damaging or deleterious effects as well as positive effects (Strawbridge, Shema, Cohen, Roberts, & Kaplan, 1998).

There is considerable variation in how individuals perceive and act on their beliefs at the end of life. Many healthcare professionals, including holistic nurses, palliative care professionals, and advocates of integrative medicine, incorporate spiritual care into their practices (Williams-Orlando, 2012). Spiritual care is one of eight domains of palliative care (National Consensus Project, 2013), and palliative care professionals have expertise in assessing and providing spiritual care at the end of life, or at least referring patients for such care. According to the Hospice and Palliative Nurses Association [HPNA] Position Statement on Spiritual Care (2010), spiritual care was foundational to Florence Nightingale's philosophy of nursing, but nevertheless, professional caregivers must not impose their own beliefs and values on patients and families (p. 2). In order to be effective, spiritual care requires nurses to recognize spirituality as being central to the human experience, the interpretation and understanding of illness, healing, health, and transcendence. It further requires the nurse to listen reflectively and to be a compassionate presence, responding to spiritual distress in patients and families, and facilitating the use of symbolism and ritual that are congruent with their preferences (Hospice and Palliative Nurses Association, 2010, p. 2).

Although hospice and palliative care professionals have expertise in holistic care for persons with serious and life-limiting illness, people die across the lifespan and across care settings. There are multiple barriers to palliative and hospice care, and many people choose not to access hospice and palliative care services during the last years of their lives. They, too, need high quality supportive care regardless of the setting, but nurses are not always comfortable providing it and are at times hampered by time constraints and other issues related to the care for dying persons. As Repenshek (2009) argues, nurses are often discomfited by moral subjectivity in end-of-life decision-making, as illustrated in Kathy's case. Lazzarrin and colleagues (2012) identified that nurses are often confronted by conflicting priorities and duties, such as the duty to follow orders and the duty to provide a comfortable death. These challenges are not always easy to overcome.

Further, nurses are frequently in a position to facilitate treatment decisions; thus, it is important for all nurses to consider the ways in which spirituality influences advance care planning; executing advance directives; life-sustaining treatment withdrawal, including artificial nutrition and hydration; and the use of advanced technology to sustain life. Both the HPNA and the American Nurses Association (ANA) have developed position statements to guide nurses in handling many of these issues (ANA Board of Directors, 2011; HPNA, 2011a, 2011c).

Spiritual Faith and Hope

Americans are for the most part religious, but there is a decline in public opinion about the influence of religion in the lives of Americans. In a religiously plural society such as the United States, the meanings and expressions of religious and spiritual faith are diverse. Recent research reveals that 9 of 10 Americans believe in God or a "higher power," and over two thirds of them use prayer as a source of comfort (Gallup & Lindsay, 1999; Okon, 2005). In addition, the percentage of Americans who indicate that religion is important to their lives has remained relatively stable over the past decade. Yet Gallup polls indicated that in 2002, 48% of survey respondents thought that the influence of religion was increasing in the United States. In 2012, only 24% of survey respondents thought it was increasing, and 72% of the respondents thought that its influence was on the decline. Between 2002 and 2012, the percentage of survey respondents who attended church dropped from 65% to 59% (Gallup, 2013).

Even if there is a decline in the influence of religion in the United States, spirituality is important to many Americans, whether or not they regularly attend religious services. In one study, the majority of respondents described themselves as being both religious and spiritual; 10 percent characterized themselves as being spiritual but nonreligious (Shahabi et al., 2002). Several studies suggest that medical professionals are less religious or spiritual than the general public. One study found that family physicians' religious and spiritual beliefs were comparable to those of the general population, but only 39 percent of psychiatrists agreed that religious faith was an important part of their lives (Bergan & Jensen, 1990). Additional studies suggest that this disparity might not be as pronounced as once thought. In sum, the extent of healthcare professionals' spiritual and religious beliefs and the influence of these beliefs in clinical decision-making have not been firmly established. Recent trends in procreative rights suggest an increasing number of pharmacists and physicians are refusing to fill and write prescriptions for what is called "Plan B," or in some cases, birth control pills. These decisions are made on the basis of religious beliefs that life begins at conception and that life must be preserved at all costs (Gee, 2006).

Even if the research on the links between religious views of healthcare professionals and practice patterns is limited, larger societal discourses surrounding the rights of living and dying in the United States have become increasingly politicized and polarized. As healthcare reform continues to be debated, highly emotionally charged and evocative expressions such as "death panels" and "pulling the plug on grandma" are commonplace, especially as states look to legislation allowing "assisted suicide." Such legislation was passed in Oregon and Washington based on the premise that persons have the right to death with dignity. Assisted suicide is not the same as active euthanasia, which involves the "act of bringing about the death of a person at his or her request" (HPNA, 2011b, p. 1). Assistive suicide requires someone to help someone who is unable to do so, commit suicide. Euthanasia is illegal in every state in the nation whereas assistive suicide is legal in about three state (Elder Law Answers, 2013). Nurses are often in the situation of being with persons who are struggling with these issues and/or spiritual distress, so it is important for nurses to develop reflective practices and be mindful of how public discourse surrounding these issues impacts the decisions that patients and their families make and/or the aftermath of decisions once they have been made. It is equally important that nurses are knowledgeable about state laws and nurse practice acts that may or may not be consistent with personal values and beliefs.

Spirituality, Risk, and Resiliency

Spiritual belief has been shown to provide social support, hope, and a mechanism to aid in coping with the fragility of life (Daugherty et al., 2004; Feher & Maly, 1999; Koenig, 2004; Taylor, 2006). In a study of the influence of spiritual beliefs in patients with advanced cancer, the authors found little association between patients' spiritual or religious problem-solving style and awareness of their prognosis or decision-making process. The study participants elected to enter the clinical trials because, in the words of one patient, "I put faith in doctors and God" (Daugherty et al., 2004, p. 141). This study found that spirituality was not associated with more or less realism about prognosis, but that it might play an important role in the patients' ability to be simultaneously realistic about poor prognoses while maintaining hope in a miracle. Similar to this study, other studies have shown that those entering clinical trials have faith in the anticancer effects of the experimental treatments, despite the low likelihood that they would be effective (Hutchinson, 1998).

Spiritual beliefs also play a significant role in deciding whether to have genetic testing. Individuals who are deeply spiritual tend to be more optimistic, more likely to attribute disease to external forces versus genetic ones, and have greater acceptance with certain diagnoses, such as cancer (Ellison & Levin, 1998; Jenkins & Pargament, 1995). In a study of women at high risk for breast cancer, the authors found that the influence of faith in genetic testing decisions, in this case BRCA1/1 testing, was dependent on a woman's perception of risk versus religious beliefs (Schwartz et al., 2000). Other studies conducted on spirituality and health risk behaviors among adolescents and pregnant women show a positive correlation between spiritual well-being and reduced health risk-taking behavior. It is important to understand the distinctions between religion and spiritual well-being. Cotton and colleagues (2005) identified that most of the adolescents in their study reported some connection with religious and spiritual concepts. Adolescents with higher levels of spiritual well-being, measured as level of existential well-being, had fewer depressive symptoms and fewer risk-taking behaviors. The authors concluded that the study supported the need to move beyond an examination of religious identification or attendance at religious services to broader concepts of spirituality (Cotton et al., 2005). Although this mechanism is not fully understood, several studies on depression in female caregivers demonstrate that religiosity was associated with feelings of "role burden" that resulted in increased symptoms of depression (Leblanc, Driscoll, & Pearlin, 2004). In addition, Pargament and colleagues (1995,) found that the use of religion as a coping mechanism, in some instances, encourages people to impose their religious views on others, to maintain interpersonal rigidity, and/or to view their suffering as something that is deserved and must be endured (Pargament, Van Haitsma, & Ensing, 1995).

The following story about Carroll offers an example of how dissonance between one's religious beliefs and behavior shape interpretations of the meaning of disease. Carroll was 38 and had three children when he confessed to his wife that he had been having sexual affairs with men. He told her that he still loved her and the children and hoped that they could stay together, but he could not keep his sexual orientation a secret any longer. His wife was devastated and could not comprehend how he could do this to her. Their religion viewed homosexuality as a sin and she asked him to go to reparative therapy to cure him. Carroll also believed that his sexual attraction to men was a sin and he agreed to enter a program. The program was not effective and Carroll was left feeling that he had failed everyone, including God. His wife divorced him and he moved from the southern town where he had been raised to live in Washington, D.C.

Ten years later, Carroll became sick and tests revealed that he was in the advanced stages of human immunodeficiency virus (HIV). He was put on five different medications to help contain the virus and prevent opportunistic infections from developing. The nurse practitioner was very clear about his need to follow the drug regimen closely and he promised that he would. He was also referred to a local HIV/AIDS community-based organization (CBO). He grew particularly close to Kathy, the same nurse in Hal's case study, who was the founder of the CBO and the volunteer "buddy" for persons living with HIV. Kathy visited Carroll frequently, and one afternoon she noticed a pile of unfilled prescriptions on his desk. When she asked why he hadn't filled them, he said that they were too expensive. She reminded him that his private insurance plan covered the cost of the medications and asked him what the real reason was. Carroll then told her that he brought this disease on himself and that it was wrong for him to use his insurance to pay for the consequences of his mistakes. There was nothing that Kathy or anyone else involved with Carroll's care could do or say to disavow him of the belief that his disease was God's retribution for his sins.

Spirituality and Individual and Familial Decision-Making

Since 1972, when the Death with Dignity Act (DDA) became law in the United States, the legal and clinical context of decision-making at the end of life has changed considerably. Both the DDA and more recent Patient Self-Determination Act of 1991 were enacted, in part, based on the assumption that power and control over life-and-death decisions should be vested in the individuals who would be most impacted by these decisions rather than professionals. Individual autonomy over choosing one's own ultimate destiny continues to be an important motivator for those completing advance directives—yet, many Americans do not have them for a variety of reasons. Deeply embedded cultural and spiritual beliefs shape individual perceptions of what constitutes a good death and who should be in charge of decision-making in regard to treatment in distinctly different ways (True et al., 2005).

Several studies have demonstrated that racial differences in advance care planning and requests for aggressive medical care in terminally ill patients exist. When compared to White individuals African Americans are less likely to have any form of advance directive and are more likely to request hospitalization and aggressive life-sustaining measures, regardless of prognosis (Caralis, Davis, Wright, & Marcial, 1993;

Johnson, Elbert-Avila, & Tulsky, 2005). These differences have been attributed to distrust of the healthcare system, economic disparities, and cultural beliefs about what constitutes "optimal" care for the dying. Although these variables are certainly valid, an individual's spiritual belief is an important variable as well (Caralis et al., 1993; Garrett, Harris, Norburn, Patrick, & Danis, 1993; Johnson et al., 2005; True et al., 2005). The following case study examines the impact of race and spiritual beliefs on the willingness of family members to forego life-sustaining treatments.

Mary was a 66-year-old African American woman with diabetes, hypertension, and early dementia who lived with her husband of 40 years. One afternoon, her husband Leonard came home to find her unconscious on the floor and called for an ambulance to take her to the hospital. An MRI showed a large arteriovenous malformation had caused an intercerebral hemorrhage and she was taken to the operating room for its repair. Although the surgeons were successful in stopping the bleeding, during the postoperative period she remained unconscious and only responded to painful stimuli by opening her eyes. When the surgeons told the husband of her poor prognosis and suggested palliative care, he refused stating, "It's in God's hands now . . . he'll take her home when he's ready." Over the next few weeks, the clinical staff became increasingly frustrated over his refusal to remove life support. They called for a palliative care consultation to help the staff work with the husband and it proved fruitful. With the assistance of Leonard's and Mary's minister, he was able to bridge hope for a miracle to the reality that she would not survive. She was taken off the ventilator and died peacefully with her husband and minister by her side.

Keeping in mind that broad generalization about any population or group is problematic, this case study supports the growing body of research about racial differences in spiritual beliefs and practices. In a comprehensive review of the literature of spirituality and end-of-life decision-making in African Americans, the authors noted four concurrent themes (Johnson et al., 2005). The first theme related to the significance of spiritual practices, particularly prayer, as a coping mechanism in times of illness. The second was related to the practice of giving their troubles to God and faith in prayer as a pathway to healing. The third theme was a belief that one's fate was in the hands of God, not man. The fourth related theme was the belief that God used physicians as an "instrument of healing" (Johnson et al., 2005). These themes are also evident in other populations, and when controlling for race and ethnicity, the most salient variable is religious faith. Interestingly, one study showed that religiosity in nurses was negatively correlated with ease in death and dying situations (Wortham, 1989). This finding, which suggests a paradox between an individual's profession of faith and trusting in God's will while clinging to artificial means to prolong life and discomfort when caring for dying patients, is interesting and worthy of much greater study. All four of these themes were present in Hal's case at the beginning of the chapter.

Although spiritual and religious beliefs are often associated with the prolongation of life-sustaining treatments, the converse is true as well. In regard to treatment preferences at the end of life, a significant barrier to hospice care among African Americans of faith is their belief that only God has the power to decide whether someone should live or die. As such, advance directives or choosing to enter a hospice program are contrary to their religious beliefs (Jackson, Schim, & Seely, 2000; Johnson et al., 2005; Reesek, Ahren, & Nair, 1999). For example, in one study participants commented that ". . . only God should end someone's suffering . . . . God is able to send cures for all illness, terminal or otherwise" (Johnson et al., 2005, p. 713). Moreover, a rare study examining nurses' attitudes toward assisted suicide revealed a positive correlation between the religiosity of nurses and a positive attitude toward assisting patients in their requests for assistance in ending their lives (Matzo, 1996). Although this study found that nurses were more inclined to discuss their decisions to assist a patient with physicians, they did not discuss them with their colleagues or supervisors. Thus we see that spiritual faith and decision-making is complex and variable and that it is important to assess individual religious views and how these are translated into clinical decision-making.

Conflicting Views: Spiritual Dissonance

Thus far, this chapter has focused primarily on the ways that spiritual beliefs are related to clinical decision-making by patients and their families. These decisions are not made in isolation, however, and often nurses are required to carry out treatments that are in contrast to their own beliefs. The following case study published in the neonatal literature offers a careful examination of the ethical and spiritual conflicts that arise between healthcare professionals and families (Stutts & Schloemann, 2002). In this scenario, a premature African American infant developed mild respiratory distress syndrome and was intubated soon after birth. Over the next several months, the infant experienced a series of complications, including severe respiratory distress, disseminated intravascular coagulation, septicemia, necrosis of the bowel, and renal failure. When the staff discussed the infant's poor prognosis with the parents, they said that the infant's ". . . outcome was in God's hands" and they refused to redirect care from aggressive to palliative intervention.

As the infant's condition continued to deteriorate, the staff grew increasingly uncomfortable with continuing aggressive therapies and asked for legal and ethical consults about their options. The hospital chaplain and members of the ethics committee spoke with the parents and as they did, the parents became more resistant and distrustful. Ultimately, the infant died 152 days after birth and the staff who cared for him went through a series of debriefing sessions. In the end, the spiritual and cultural conflicts that arose between the staff and parents made it difficult for the professionals to provide what they believed to be optimal care for the infant. Although the debriefing sessions were useful, the authors conclude by emphasizing how the situation might have been prevented if the staff had spent more time considering the situation through the social, cultural, and spiritual lens of the parents (Stutts & Schloemann, 2002).

In this scenario, the professionals viewed issues of bioethics and quality of life quite differently than the parents. The resultant dissonance resulted in the parents becoming increasingly defensive and suspicious of the professionals. At the same time, the staff became increasingly anguished about having to prolong what they perceived to be suffering in the infant. In this case, the hospital was proactive in supporting the staff by providing time to debrief and express their frustration in an open and nonjudgmental manner. Although these group meetings did not totally diffuse the situation, they did provide a venue for the staff to receive support and express their concerns. This case study reveals how disparate views about the appropriate care of terminally ill children impact the experiences of dying and loss. The staff did not fully understand the deep and profound sense of loss the parents were experiencing. Although the staff dealt with these issues on a daily basis and desired to end the infant's suffering, the parents were naïve to such situations. Professional discussions of medical futility and explanations of the findings of ethics committees did little to support them and, in fact, served to alienate the parents. In trying to do what the staff deemed best for the infant, they failed to provide the type of supportive care the parents needed during this time of crisis. If they had fully considered the parents' perspective and responded accordingly, they might well have been able to help the parents in their grief.

Moral Distress and Decision-Making Among Professionals

It is important for healthcare professionals to consider another person's point of view. It is equally important that they reflect upon their own beliefs. Many times intra- and interprofessional and interpersonal conflicts arise but the true source of the conflict is never identified. In the case studies presented so far in this chapter, difficulties arise when there is a dissonance between patient and family values and worldviews and those of health professionals. The extant literature on the role of faith in medical decision-making among health professionals suggests that faith is not an important factor in physician and nurse decision-making

(Okon, 2005). Still, as we saw in the neonatal case study, nurses often experience "moral distress" when they are required to act in a manner that violates personal beliefs and values about what is right and wrong (Fenton, 1988; Houghtaling, 2012; McAndrew, Leske, & Garcia, 2011; Weigand & Funk, 2012). Moral distress has been found to be a significant source of emotional suffering in nurses and anecdotally associated with job dissatisfaction and decreased quality patient care, and implicated in nurses leaving the workforce (Nathaniel, 2002).

A growing body of literature examining the source and manifestations of moral distress in nurses demonstrates that the continuation of futile care often evokes strong emotional responses from nurses (Ferrell, 2006). Psychologists define moral distress as the state experienced when moral choices and actions are thwarted by constraints (Austin, Rankel, Kagan, Bergum, & Lemermeyer, 2005). Moral dilemmas among nurses arise due to a variety of factors, including institutional demands, interpersonal and intraprofessional conflicts, and interdisciplinary disputes (Lazzarin et al., 2012; McAndrew et al., 2011; Weigand & Funk, 2012). The intensity of moral distress and the work environment have been linked to the frequency of moral distress experienced by nurses. One study suggests a negative correlation between age and moral distress intensity, and that being African American was related to higher levels of moral distress intensity (Corley, Minick, Elswick, & Jacobs, 2005). In critical care nurses, the frequency of moral distress situations that are perceived as futile or unbeneficial to their patients has a significant relationship to the experience of emotional exhaustion, a main component of burnout (Meltzer & Huckabay, 2004). Thus, it behooves health professionals to critically examine the sources and implications of moral distress in the clinical arena and to develop preventive measures, as well as interventions to reduce the negative effects of moral distress when it occurs.

Moral distress among nurses has far-reaching implications. Moral distress adversely affects job satisfaction, retention, psychological and physical well-being, self-image, and spirituality. Experience of moral distress also influences attitudes toward the nurse's execution of personal advance directives and participation in blood donation and organ donation. Critical care and emergency department nurses commonly encounter situations that are associated with high levels of moral distress, and the impact of this distress has implications that extend well beyond job satisfaction and retention (Houghtaling, 2012; Weigand & Funk, 2012). In sum, it is imperative that strategies to mitigate moral distress in nurses are developed and resources allocated to create an organizational culture that supports nurses who are experiencing moral or spiritual distress related to patient care.

Given the complexities of the healthcare system today, and the profound and lingering effects of choosing to assist individuals in dying, whether tacitly or actively, it is important to critically examine these issues and provide opportunities for nurses working with persons with progressive and serious illness and their families to meet with supportive colleagues. By providing a safe environment where nurses can share their experiences with troubling cases and moral conflict, lasting effects of moral distress such as burnout and substance abuse might be avoided.

Spirituality, Nursing, and Decision-Making: Where to Go from Here?

Thus far, this chapter has examined the influence of morals, values, and spirituality on decision-making from the perspectives of patients, families, and health professionals. A series of case studies were used to help explore the complexities and often paradoxical links between religious belief and end-of-life decision-making. What is clear from these case studies is that although groups of people might share a common set of religious tenets and beliefs, each individual's perceptions of the meaning of these beliefs and how they should be acted upon differ considerably within the group. Spiritual faith is not static; it changes in the contexts of time and experience. Moreover, one's spirituality is often influenced by a dynamic interaction among social, cultural, physical, and psychological factors that shade one's perception and interpretation of life events. For example, even though an individual might execute an advance directive when he or she is healthy, in the face of acute illness, that individual might well change their mind and request aggressive therapies that might or might not be appropriate. Even those who have deep spiritual faith can be fearful in the face of death.

There is a growing body of literature in the role of religion and spirituality in individual and familial end-of-life decision-making. This literature reveals a dissonance among the needs of medical institutions, health professionals, and the seriously and critically ill. In the 1970s, the ethics literature was full of compelling testimonials of those who believed their loved ones were terminally ill. In one case, the parents of a premature infant wrote that their dying infant was "entrapped in an intensive care unit where the machinery is [was] more sophisticated than the code of law and ethics governing its use" (Stinson & Stinson, 1981, p. 5). More currently, as Kirschbaum (1996) points out, the ethics literature "has swung to describe parents' demands for futile treatment as autonomy gone wild" (p. 51). There is ample evidence of the increasing conflict between the religious convictions of patients and their families and professional clinical decision-making (Brett & Jersild, 2003). Although the literature on interventions to help healthcare professionals and patients' families to reframe their convictions in ways that might be mutually beneficial is sparse, it does exist (Brett & Jersild, 2003; Okon, 2005; Sessanna et al., 2010). As noted in the neonatal intensive care case study, there were things that the staff could have done to promote a more positive outcome for the parents. Although the loss of an infant is devastating, if the staff understood the complexities of the parents' reactions, listened carefully to their concerns, and viewed the situation from their perspective, the results might have been quite different.

Over the past 10 years, myriad tools and resources have been made publically available to help nurses and the general public to understand and measure spirituality and to develop spiritual care expertise. Both HPNA and the National Consensus Project's Clinical Guidelines for Quality Palliative Care provide evidence-based guidance on best practices related to spiritual care (HPNA, 2013; National Consensus Project, 2013). Okon (2005) and Sessanna and colleagues (2011) provide comprehensive reviews of the spiritual aspects of palliative care, details of the various instruments used in clinical research, assessment tools, approaches to conducting spiritual histories from religious and existential perspectives, and effective communication techniques. Interventions such as unit-based training in spirituality have improved the quality of care in progressive care units (Lind, Sendelbach, & Steen, 2011). Regardless of the tools that are used as a basis for assessment and discussion, a few principles should be considered.

Although there is debate over the appropriate role for nurses in providing spiritual care for their patients (van Leeuwen et al., 2006), it is clear that nurses' spiritual and religious beliefs shape their interactions with their colleagues and patients. Although some nurses are comfortable discussing spiritual concerns with patients and their families when they arise, many nurses are not. The Working Group on Religious and Spiritual Issues at the End of Life has set guidelines in regard to health professionals attending to the spiritual needs of patients. The guidelines encourage listening carefully to patients and to show respect for their views, but to avoid theological discussions unless having the requisite training to do so and this is requested by the patient. The guidelines also suggest that appropriate professional resources should be used to support the patient, such as a referral to a chaplain or, as in Mary and Leonard's case, the patient's minister or parish nurse.

The case studies in this chapter highlight real-life exemplars of the interrelationships between spirituality beliefs and practices and clinical decision-making. When confronted with issues of living and dying, each person comes with their unique perspective and handles these issues in their own time and in their own way. Although there are guides available to assist nurses, it is important to remember this when working with patients and their families. Nurses can best support each other, patients, and their families if they reflect on their own spirituality while listening carefully and respecting the views of others.

References

Amenta, M. O. R. (1984). Traits of hospice nurses compared with those who work in traditional setting. *Journal of Clinical Psychology, 40*(2), 414–420.

American Nurses Association Board of Directors. (2011). *Position statement: Forgoing nutrition and hydration.* Accessed March 2, 2013, from http://www.nursingworld.org/MainMenuCategories/EthicsStandards/Ethics-Position-Statements/prtetnutr14451.aspx

American Heritage (1992). *American Heritage dictionary of the English language,* (3rd ed.). Boston: Houghton-Mifflin.

Antonovsky, A. (1979). *Health, stress, and coping.* San Francisco: Jossey-Bass Publishers.

Antonovsky, A. (1987). *Unraveling the mystery of health.* San Francisco: Jossey-Bass Publishers.

Austin, W., Rankel, M., Kagan, L., Bergum, V., & Lemermeyer, G. (2005). To stay or to go, to speak or stay silent, to act or not to act: Moral distress as experienced by psychologists. *Ethics and Behavior, 15*(3), 197–212.

Bergan, A. E., & Jensen, J. P. (1990). Religiosity of psychotherapists: A national survey. *Psychotherapy, 27*, 3–7.

Brett, A., & Jersild, P. (2003). "Inappropriate" treatment near the end of life: Conflict between religious convictions and clinical judgment. *Archives of Internal Medicine, 163*, 1645–1649.

Buck, J. (2004). Home health versus home hospice: Cooperation, competition and co-optation. *Nursing History Review, 12*, 25–46.

Buck, J. (2005). *Rights of passage: Reforming care for the dying, 1965–1986.* Charlottesville: University of Virginia.

Buck, J. (2006). "Manna from heaven": Religion, nursing, and the modern hospice concept. *Windows in Time, 14*(1), 6–9.

Buck, J. (2007). Reweaving a tapestry of care: Nursing, religion and the meaning of hospice, 1945–1978. *Nursing History Review, 15*, 113–145.

Buck, J. (2010). Nursing the borderlands of life: Hospice and the politics of health care reform. In S. Lewenson & P. D'Antonio (Eds.), *Nursing history: Interventions through time* (pp. 201–220). New York: Springer Publishing Company.

Buck, J. (2011). Policy and the reformation of hospice: Lessons from the past to guide the future of palliative care. *Journal of Hospice and Palliative Nursing, 13*(6), S35–S43. doi: 10.1097/NJH.0b013e3182331160.

Buhler-Wilkerson, K. (2001). *No place like home: A history of nursing and home care in the United States.* Baltimore: The Johns Hopkins University Press.

Caralis, P., Davis, B., Wright, K., & Marcial, E. (1993). The influence of ethnicity and race on attitudes toward advance directives, life-prolonging treatments, and euthanasia. *Journal of Clinical Ethics, 4*, 155–165.

Cassel, E. (1974). Death in a technological society. In P. Steifels & R. Veatch (Eds.), *The Hastings Center report: Death inside out.* New York: Harper & Row.

Clark, D. (1997). Someone to watch over me . . . Cicely Saunders. *Nursing Times, 93*(34), 50–52.

Clark, D. (1998). Originating a movement: Cicely Saunders and the development of St. Christopher's Hospice, 1957–1967. *Mortality, 3*(1), 43–63.

Corley, M. C., Minick, P., Elswick, R. K., & Jacobs, M. (2005). Nurse moral distress and ethical work environment. *Nursing Ethics, 12*(4), 381–390.

Cotton, S., Larkin, E., Hoopes, A., Cromer, B. A., & Rosenthal, S. L. (2005). The impact of adolescent spirituality on depressive symptoms and health risk behaviors. *Journal of Adolescent Health, 36*(6), 472–480.

Daugherty, C., Fitchett, G., Murphy, P., Peterman, A., Banik, D., Hlubocky, F., et al. (2004). Trusting God and medicine: Spirituality in advanced cancer patients volunteering for clinical trials of experimental agents. *Psycho-Oncology, 14*, 135–146.

du Boulay, S. (1984). *Cicely Saunders, founder of the modern hospice movement*. New York: Amaryllis Press.

Duff, R., & Hollingshead, A. (1968). *Sickness and society*. New York: Harper & Row.

Elder Law Answers (2013). Retrieved from http://www.elderlawanswers.com/is-assisted-suicide-legal-9921

Ellison, C. G., & Levin, J. S. (1998). The religion-health connection: Evidence, theory, and future directions. *Health Education Behavior, 25*, 700–720.

Feher, S., & Maly, R. (1999). Coping with breast cancer in later life: The role of religious faith. *Psycho-Oncology, 8*, 408–416.

Fenton, M. (1988). Moral distress in clinical practice: Implications for the nurse administrator. *Canadian Journal of Nursing Administration, 1*, 8–11.

Ferrell, B. R. (2006). Journal club. Understanding the moral distress of nurses witnessing medically futile care. *Oncology Nursing Forum, 33*(5), 922–930.

Filene, P. (1998). *In the arms of others: A cultural history of the right to die in America*. Chicago: Ivan R. Dee.

Gallup. (2013). *Gallup poll on historical trends in religion in the United States*. Retrieved from http://www.gallup.com/poll/1690/religion.aspx

Gallup, G., & Lindsay, D. (1999). *Surveying the religious landscape: Trends in U.S. beliefs*. Harrisburg, PA: Morehouse Publishing.

Garrett, J., Harris, R., Norburn, J., Patrick, D., & Danis, M. (1993). Life-sustaining treatments during terminal illness: Who wants what? *Journal of General Internal Medicine, 8*, 361–368.

Gee, R. (2006). Plan B, reproductive rights, and physician activism. *New England Journal of Medicine, 355*(1), 4–5.

Glaser, B., & Strauss, A. (1965). *Awareness of dying*. Chicago: Aldine Press.

Glaser, B., & Strauss, A. (1968). *Time for dying*. Chicago: Aldine Press.

Hospice and Palliative Nurses Association (2010). *HPNA position statement: Spiritual care*. Retrieved from https://www.hpna.org/DisplayPage.aspx?Title=Position%20Statements

Hospice and Palliative Nurses Association (2011a). *HPNA position statement: Artificial nutrition and hydration in advanced illness*. Retrieved from https://www.hpna.org/DisplayPage.aspx?Title=Position%20Statements

Hospice and Palliative Nurses Association (2011b). *HPNA position statement: Legalization of assisted suicide*. Retrieved from https://www.hpna.org/DisplayPage.aspx?Title=Position%20Statements

Hospice and Palliative Nurses Association (2011c). *HPNA position statement: Withholding and/or withdrawing life-sustaining therapies*. Retrieved from https://www.hpna.org/DisplayPage.aspx?Title=Position%20Statements

Houghtaling, D. (2012). Moral distress: An invisible challenge for trauma nurses. *Journal of Trauma Nursing, 19*(4), 232–237. doi: 10.1097/JTN.0b013e318261d2dc.

Humphreys, C. (2001). "Waiting for the last summons": The establishment of the first hospices in England, 1878–1914. *Mortality, 6*(2), 146–166.

Hutchinson, C. (1998). Phase I trials in cancer patients: Participants' perceptions. *European Journal of Cancer Care, 7*, 15–22.

Jackson, F., Schim, S., & Seely, S. (2000). Barriers to hospice care for African Americans: Problems and solutions. *Journal of Hospice and Palliative Nursing, 2*, 65–72.

Jenkins, R. A., & Pargament, K. (1995). Religion and spirituality as resources for coping with cancer. *Journal of Psychosocial Oncology, 13*, 51–74.

Johnson, K., Elbert-Avila, K., & Tulsky, J. (2005). The influence of spiritual beliefs and practices in the treatment preferences of African Americans: A review of the literature. *Journal of the American Geriatrics Society, 53*, 711–719.

Kirschbaum, M. S. (1996). Life support decisions for children: What do parents value? *Advances in Nursing Science, 19*(1), 51–71.

Koenig, H. (2004). Religion, spirituality, and medicine: Research findings and implications for clinical practice. *Southern Medical Journal, 97*(12), 1194–2000.

Krisman-Scott, M. A. (2001). Origins of hospice in the United States: The care of the dying, 1945–1975. *Journal of Hospice and Palliative Nursing, 5*(4), 205–212.

Kübler-Ross, E. (1969). *On death and dying*. New York: Macmillan House.

Lazzarin, M., Biondi, A., & Di Mauro, S. (2012). Moral distress in nurses in oncology and haematology units. *Nursing Ethics, 19*(2), 183–195. doi: 10.1177/0969733011416840.

Leblanc, A. J., Driscoll, A. K., & Pearlin, L. I. (2004). Religiosity and the expansion of caregiver stress. *Aging and Mental Health, 8*(5), 410–421.

Lind, B., Sendelbach, S., & Steen, S. (2011). Effects of a spirituality training program for nurses on patients in a progressive care unit. *Critical Care Nurse, 31*(3), 87–90.

Matzo, M. L. (1996). *Registered nurses' attitudes toward and practices of assisted suicide and patient-requested euthanasia* (Unpublished doctoral dissertation). University of Massachusetts at Boston.

McAndrew, N., Leske, J., & Garcia, A. (2011). Influence of moral distress on the professional practice environment during prognostic conflict in critical care. *Journal of Trauma Nursing, 18*(4), 221–230. doi: 10.1097/JTN.0b013e31823a4a12.

McSherry, W., & Cash, K. (2004). The language of spirituality: An emerging taxonomy. *International Journal of Nursing Studies, 41*, 151–161.

Meltzer, L. S., & Huckabay, L. M. (2004). Critical care nurses' perceptions of futile care and its effect on burnout. *American Journal of Critical Care, 13*(3), 202–208.

Merriam-Webster (2003). *Merriam-Webster's collegiate dictionary* (11th ed.). Springfield, MA: Merriam-Webster.

Nathaniel, A. (2002). Moral distress among nurses. *The American Nurses Association Ethics and Humane Rights Issues Update, 1*(3), 1–8.

National Consensus Project for Quality Palliative Care (2013). *Clinical practice guidelines for quality palliative care* (3rd ed.). Retrieved from http://www.nationalconsensusproject.org

O'Brien, M. E. (1999). *Spirituality in nursing: Standing on holy ground.* London: Jones & Bartlett Publishers International.

Okon, T. (2005). Spiritual, religious, and existential aspects of palliative care. *Journal of Palliative Medicine, 8*(2), 392–419.

Pannier, E. (1980). *The hospice caregiver: A qualitative study*. Evanston, IL: Northwestern University Press.

Pargament, K. L., Van Haitsma, K. S., & Ensing, D. S. (1995). Religion in coping. In M. A. Kimble, S. H. McFadden, J. W. Ellor, & J. J. Seeber (Eds.), *Aging, spirituality, and religion: A handbook* (pp. 47–49). Minneapolis, MN: Fortress Press.

Post-White, J., Ceronsky, C., Kreitzer, M., Nickelson, K., Drew, D., Mackey, K. W., et al. (1996). Hope, spirituality, sense of coherence, and quality of life in patients with cancer. *Oncology Nursing Forum, 23*(10), 1571–1579.

Quint, J. (1967). *The nurse and the dying patient.* New York: Macmillan.

Reesek, D. J., Ahren, R. E., & Nair, S. (1999). Hospice access and use by African Americans: Addressing cultural and institutional barriers through participatory action research. *Social Work, 44*, 549–559.

Repenshek, M. (2009). Moral distress: Inability to act or discomfort with moral subjectivity? *Nursing Ethics, 16*(6), 734–742. doi: 10.1177/0969733009342138.

Schwartz, M., Hughes, C., Roth, J., Main, D., Peshkin, B., Isaacs, C., et al. (2000). Spiritual faith and genetic testing decisions among high-risk breast cancer probands. *Cancer Epidemiology, Biomarkers and Prevention, 9*, 381–385.

Sessanna, D., Finnell, M., Underhill, Y., & Peng, H. (2011). Measures assessing spirituality as more than religiosity: A methodological review of nursing and health-related literature. *Journal of Advanced Nursing, 67*(8), 1677–1694. doi: 10.1111/j.1365-2648.2010.05596.x.

Shahabi, L., Powell, L., Musick, M., Pargament, K., Thoresen, C., & Williams, D. (2002). Correlates of self-perceptions of spirituality in American adults. *Annals of Behavioral Medicine, 24*, 59–68.

Shelley, J., & Miller, A. B. (1999). *Called to care: A Christian theology of nursing.* Downers Grove, IL: InterVarsity Press.

Siebold, C. (1992). *The hospice movement: Easing death's pain.* New York: Twayne Publishers.

Smith, S., & Nickel, D. (1999). From home to hospital: Parallels in birthing and dying in twentieth-century Canada. *Canadian Bulletin of Medical History, 16*(1), 49–64.

Stinson, R., & Stinson, P. (1981). On the death of a baby. *Journal of Medical Ethics, 7*, 5–18.

Strawbridge, W. J., Shema, S. J., Cohen, R. D., Roberts, R. E., & Kaplan, G. A. (1998). Religiosity buffers effects of some stressors on depression but exacerbates others. *Journals of Gerontology Series B: Psychological Sciences and Social Sciences, 53*(3), S118–S126.

Stutts, A., & Schloemann, J. (2002). Life-sustaining support: Ethical, cultural and spiritual conflicts, Part II: Staff support—A neonatal case study. *Neonatal Network, 21*(4), 27–34.

Sudnow, D. (1967). *Passing on: The social organization of dying*. Upper Saddle River, NJ: Prentice Hall.

Tanyi, R. (2002). Toward clarification of the meaning of spirituality. *Journal of Advanced Nursing, 39*(5), 500–509.

Taylor, E. J. (2006). Prevalence and associated factors of spiritual needs among patients with cancer and family caregivers. *Oncology Nursing Forum, 33*(4), 729–735.

True, G., Phipps, E., Braitman, L., Harralson, T., Harris, D., & Tester, W. (2005). Treatment preferences and advance care planning at end of life: The role of ethnicity and spiritual coping in cancer patients. *Annals of Behavioral Medicine, 30*(2), 174–179.

van Leeuwen, R., Tiesinga, L., Post, D., & Jochemsen, H. (2006). Spiritual care: Implications for nurses' professional responsibility. *Journal of Clinical Nursing, 15*(7), 875–884.

Walsh, J. (1929). *The history of nursing*. New York: PJ Kennedy and Sons.

Webb, M. (1997). *The good death: The new American search to reshape the end of life*. New York: Bantam Books.

Weigand, D., & Funk, M. (2012). Consequences of clinical situations that cause critical care nurses to experience moral distress. *Nursing Ethic, 19*(4), 479–487. doi: 10.1177/0969733011429342.

Williams-Orlando, C. (2012). Spirituality in integrative medicine. *Integrative Medicine, 11*(4), 34–39.

Wortham, C. B. (1989). *An investigation of the influence of religiosity on the ease with which nurses respond to death and dying situations*. Atlanta: Emory University Press.

Chapter 5

Culture and Decision-Making

Caroline Camuñas

Decision-making is a complex process. It involves gathering and making sense of a great deal of information; culture makes up a large part of that information. The culture of individuals, families, groups, organizations, and the population impacts the quality of our decisions and their outcomes. Astute, knowledgeable, considered application of culture theory is essential for effective, appropriate decisions. As nursing leaders we have learned the importance of making such on-target decisions to improve the quality of care, work relationships, and the myriad of outcomes. This chapter explores the meaning of culture and its influence on the decisions that we make, and includes case studies to help clarify the various ideas and concepts about this influence.

Culture

Culture has various definitions. The discipline of philosophy defines culture as the way of life of a people, including their attitudes, values, beliefs, arts, sciences, modes of perception, and habits of thought and activity. Cultural features are learned but are often too pervasive to be readily noticed from within (Blackburn, 1996). Anthropologist Margaret Meade understood culture to mean "the systematic body of learned behavior which is transmitted from parents to children" (Macklin, 1999, p. 6). In terms of nursing, Leininger (2002) defined culture as "patterned lifeways, values, beliefs, norms, symbols, and practices of individuals, groups, or institutions that are learned, shared, and usually transmitted intergenerationally over time" (p. 83). Purnell and Paulanka (2012) further described culture as the totality of socially transmitted behavioral patterns, arts, beliefs, values, customs, lifeways, and all other products of human work and thought characteristics of a population of people that guide their worldview and decision-making. Another definition of culture important to nurses is one used by business. Organizational culture is important in the business world and is defined as the pattern of role-related beliefs, values, and expectations that is shared by members of an organization (Dickson, 1994). These patterns produce the rules and norms of behavior that have a powerful influence on individual and group behavior within the organization. A person's role-related values include both personal values and organizational values. See **Table 5-1** to understand how an individual's personal values relate to the values within an organizational culture (Dickson, 1994).

Organizational culture impacts all individuals in an organization, whether patients, nurses, or other employees. The healthcare environment in which one works influences the "opportunities, values, commitment, satisfaction, and motivation" of nurses (Jeffries, 2010, p. 254). Porter O'Grady and Malloch (2011) explain that organizational culture often covertly and subtly impacts the decisions made within an organization. The culture of that organization also impacts the "leadership styles" and strategies that are formulated for "organizational change" (p. 363). An important example of this organizational culture is the culture shock nurses suffer when their values conflict with those of the organization in which they work, as identified in Kramer's seminal work in the early 1970s (Kramer, 1974; Kramer & Schmalenberg, 1977). Culture shock is turmoil or a disturbance of mental equilibrium that includes feelings of helplessness, powerlessness, frustration, and dissatisfaction when a new culture or subculture is encountered. Attempts are made to understand and effectively adapt to the different group or practice. It can also be experienced in one's own culture when a new or novel event or circumstance takes place. Any and all who come in contact with the healthcare system can experience culture shock.

Cultural diversity includes differences in race, ethnicity, national origin, religion, age, gender, sexual orientation, ability or disability, social and economic status or class, education, and other such traits of groups of people (Andrews & Boyle, 2012). For example, this may

Table 5-1

Organizational Culture: Shared Values

Personal Values	Role-Related Values	Organizational Values
Ambition	Ambition	Leadership in care and science
Beneficence	Beneficence	Beneficence, excellence
Compassion	Compassion	Service quality
Courage	Patient satisfaction	Patient satisfaction
Excellence	Excellence	Improved decision-making
Fairness, justice	Competence	Internal competition
Family	Ingenuity, creativity	External competition
Honesty, truth	Honesty, truth	Honesty, truth
Independence	Resourcefulness	Innovation
Integrity	Integrity	Efficiency and cost control
Loyalty	Shared goals	Shared goals
Nonmaleficence	Nonmaleficence	Nonmaleficence
Respect for autonomy	Respect for autonomy	Respect for employee and patient autonomy
Responsibility	Responsibility	Responsibility

Source: Marketing management by Dickson, Peter R. Reproduced with permission of Dryden Press in the format Republish in a book via Copyright Clearance Center.

be exemplified by immigrant or minority families and groups and includes individual families that have their own blend of group and personal characteristics. Within each family, individuals have their own beliefs, hopes, strengths, weaknesses, limitations, and goals—special group and personal characteristics developed over generations through shared history. Ignoring important aspects of cultural diversity have led to major disparities in health care. The literature shows research evidence that demonstrates prevalent race and gender discrimination in healthcare allocation (Bach, Pham, Schrag, Tate, & Hargraves, 2004; Bloche, 2004; Haiman et al., 2006; Jeffries, 2010; Smedley, Stith, & Nelson, 2003; Steinbrook, 2004). Subsequent research continues to support these findings (National Research Council and Institute of Medicine, 2013). Such evidence shows that culture has often been absent from decision-making regarding the planning, implementation, and evaluation of our healthcare system.

Healthcare providers increasingly encounter persons from diverse cultures. The population of the United States is becoming more diverse; although all minority groups are growing, some, such as Hispanics, are growing faster than others. It is not too difficult to foresee a future in which every group is a minority. Although minority groups are growing, that growth is not yet reflected in the nursing workforce (see **Table 5-2**). This may well portend the need, now more than ever, to prepare culturally competent nurses. Jeffries's (2010) definition of cultural competence reads as a clear directive for nurse educators and nurses. Cultural competence is a "multidimensional learning process that integrates transcultural nursing skills in all three dimensions of learning (cognitive, practical, and affective), involves transcultural self-efficacy (confidence) as a major influencing factor and aims to achieve culturally congruent nursing care" (Jeffries, 2010, p. 46).

Leininger and McFarland (2006) affirm that nursing is a unique caring profession that serves others around the world, and that nursing is affected by ethnohistory, culture, social structures, environmental factors in varied areas, and the different needs of people. In order to practice competently, nurses must include technological, religious, philosophical, kinship and social connections, cultural values and lifeways, and political, legal, economic, educational, and any other pertinent factors that influence health and well-being. These factors are all part of Leininger's

Table 5-2

Diversity: U.S. Population and Nurse Population, 2010

	Total Population	Percentage of Population	Nurses	Percentage of Nurses
United States	308,745,538	100	3,036,162	100
White	223,538,285	72.4	2,526,087	83.2
Black	38,901,938	12.6	1,639,528	5.4
Hispanic	50,325,523	16.3	109,302	3.6
Asian	14,819,786	4.8		
American Indian/Alaska Native	2,778,710	0.9	9,109	0.3
Native Hawaiian/Pacific Islander	617,491	0.2	176,097[1]	5.8[2]
Other	8,953,621	2.9	516,148[3]	1.7

Note: Total population percentage more than 100 percent due to rounding.
[1, 2] Asian included with Native Hawaiian/Pacific Islander in 2010 data.
[3] Two or more races, non-Hispanic in 2010 data.

Source: US Census Bureau, Census 2010, Summary File 1 and USDHHS, Health Resource and Service Administration September 2010.

seminal Sunshine Model, which can be used in decision-making. This knowledge is necessary to help people with their diverse care needs.

Analysis of these factors or influencers led Leininger (2002) to identify three main actions and decision guides to provide safe, culturally congruent, and meaningful health care to those of a different culture from one's own. These guides were: (1) culture care preservation and/or maintenance, (2) culture care accommodation and/or negotiation, and (3) culture care repatterning and/or restructuring. The reader is directed to works by Leininger and McFarland (2006) and Jeffries (2010) for a more in-depth discussion about culturally competent care and transcultural nursing.

Patterns of Knowing

Culture is a part of the body of knowledge that nurses use to provide care. As a result, when considering this body of knowledge and its effect on the decisions nurses make, understanding patterns of knowing informs this process. This section explores the evolution of meaning behind patterns of knowing and its connections to Leininger's (2002) cultural guides.

In her seminal study, Carper (1978) identified that the patterns, forms, and structures of knowledge nurses use in practice consist of (1) empirics, (2) esthetics, (3) ethics or moral knowledge, and (4) personal knowledge. *Empirics*, or the science of nursing, is concerned with describing, explaining, and predicting phenomena. *Esthetics*, or the art of nursing, is the expressive and perceptive aspect of nursing that is little understood. *Ethics* is philosophy regarding morality and focuses on right and wrong, good and bad. It is about the "why" of morality, and attempts to explicate or answer why something is right or wrong, good or bad. Nursing has a "high expectation for moral integrity," and nurses' personal values and beliefs influence this expectation (Ebby et al., 2013, p. 229). *Personal knowledge* ". . . is concerned with the knowing, encountering, and actualizing of the concrete, individual self" (Carper, 1978, p. 18).

Science is the method through which knowledge of human beings and the world is organized. Factors such as intuition, experience, and good judgment contribute to new knowledge in science (Chernow & Vallasi, 1993, p. 2452). Rogers (1988) asserted that it is through "the imaginative and creative use of knowledge that nurses can know and understand the health care needs of people" (p. 10). Knowledge development and research are generally embedded in cultural values and perspectives. We study what is important to us; what is important to us generally has a cultural base (Ketefian & Redman, 1977).

Johnson (1994), in a dialectical study, identified the following five distinct conceptualizations that can be identified as art or the esthetic knowing in nursing: (1) grasping meaning in patient encounters, (2) establishing a meaningful connection with the patient, (3) performing nursing activities skillfully, (4) determining an appropriate course of action rationally, and (5) conducting one's nursing practice ethically. Understanding meaning is essential; attention must be paid to experience. Lack of attention to experience is a disservice to patients and can put them at risk. Chinn and Kramer (1991) understand esthetic knowing as what makes it possible to know what to do in a given moment, instantly, without conscious deliberation (p. 10).

Carper (1978) acknowledged that personal knowledge is the "most problematic, the most difficult to master and to teach" (p. 18). Self-awareness is a dynamic and transformative process that is essential to understanding the person (patient) before you. Interpersonal relationships, interactions, and transactions are intrinsic to nursing. This process is of primary concern in a healing relationship (Eckroth-Bucher, 2010). Personal knowing requires that you are in relationship with the human being as a person. There must be an openness, a freedom from categories, classifications, and pigeonholes. We must be in a relationship that is not generalized by beliefs, concepts, expectations, and stereotypes. In doing so, we have to be willing and able to accept ambiguity, vagueness, and discrepancy of others and ourselves. Jeffries (2010), for example, refers to the need for faculty in an academic setting to begin educating learners about transcultural nursing by starting with a self-assessment. By doing a systematic assessment of the various cultural dimensions that may influence decisions during the teaching–learning process, nurses put into action the meaning of knowing and self-awareness.

Ethics is the fourth pattern of knowing identified by Carper (1978). Moral discomfort and moral dilemmas arise in situations of uncertainty and ambiguity. Nonmaleficence and beneficence are principles basic to nursing practice, along with the principles of respect for autonomy and justice. Beyond principles is care and caring or care-based ethics, which is another approach to understanding moral life. Care has developed as a theory of ethics that is important in private life (family and friends) as well as in public life (law, medical, and nursing practice; politics; the organization of society; war; and international relations). Care-based ethics is concerned with *how* we do what we do. Cameron-Traub (2002) refers to the importance of cultural systems or codes "that guide societal caring and maintain the social fabric, for example, by limiting injustices that are inconsistent with sociability, and social well-being" (p. 169). Nurses, when making decisions, must take into account these guides as well as the "differences and similarities, or universals, in moral and ethical aspects of care and caring" (Cameron-Taub, 2002, p. 169).

The following case study examines the author's experience in working with a student who learned how to negotiate between her own culture and that of the educational organization.

Case Study 1

Some time ago I received an e-mail from an Asian nurse with whom I had worked as a leader on a teaching project in Vietnam with Health Volunteers Overseas (HVO). Lisa was studying at a U.S. university and developing her research to earn a doctorate. In her "SOS" message she said she had begun to work with a professor, but the fit with her project was not the best. Another professor whose ideas and work converged with her own had suddenly become available. Lisa asked if it was acceptable to change sponsors. Her U.S. classmates encouraged her to talk with her sponsor. Colleagues from her homeland told her not to; they would be mad if someone did this to them.

I wrote to Lisa and advised her to talk with her sponsor and explain to her what she had explained to me and ask her to approve the change. Lisa did so and then changed sponsors with no hard feelings. By negotiating a path between two cultures, Lisa was able to satisfy her learning needs and achieve success. In this environment, she had become bicultural.

Care, Caring, and Culture

In health care, we talk about care in several ways. First, care is understood as physical, as in taking care of or doing something for another; it is an activity. The second sense of care is to use caution or to be careful to do something correctly in order to avoid accident, injury, or hurt. These two meanings have to do with the cognitive and psychomotor domains in education. The third sense of care deals with emotion and attitude, as in caring about something, and falls within the affective domain. Beauchamp and Childress (2009) and Barnum (1998) assert that the expression of caring makes a critical difference. When caring is absent, nurses can fail patients in important ways. Emotional engagement and communication are important parts of human relationships in general, and health care in particular, and both require a level of cultural competence in order to meet the needs of those being cared for, whether an individual, family, community, or group.

Leininger (2002) wrote about her earlier seminal ideas about the "universality of culture care" and the "diversity of culture care," explaining that nurses needed to learn about the individual and group differences and "respond to such variabilities" (p. 73). Leininger further explains that:

> Transculturally, there are many different ways of knowing that go beyond empirical, personal, aesthetic or ethical nursing theories. Cultures influence and shape ways of knowing and explaining that may be religious (spiritual), materialistic, technological, experiential, and culture–value based theories. (p. 73)

As we explore the meaning of knowing, caring, and culture, we recognize that a great many factors go into the decisions that are made, and that culture is embedded in every decision.

Unknowing

These fundamental patterns discussed above are important in the consideration of culture, care, and decision-making. Yet, they are not the whole of knowing. Munhall (1993) identified and explicated how unknowing is important for nurses because it makes them authentically present for the patient. Unknowing is essential to understanding the intersubjective and the perspective. Munhall asserts that it is "essential that we understand our self and our patient to be two distinctive beings, one of whom we do not know" (p. 125). Intersubjectivity is the verbal and nonverbal influence between the organized subjective world of one person and the organized subjective world of another. It is within this intersubjective field that caring, understanding, empathy, conflict, and misunderstandings occur (p. 126). Unknowing, then, is a condition of openness; it allows persons to be. It is "the actual essence of the meaning an experience has for a patient" (p. 128). As such, unknowing plays a role in how decisions are made, especially when considering delivering culturally competent care.

In-Between and Beyond

Silva, Sorrell, and Sorrell (1995) critiqued Carper's patterns of knowing and identified strengths and weaknesses. Their work grows from a shift in worldview or philosophy. A major contribution made by Carper was that she helped nurses understand that how we come to know is "complex, diverse, ever emerging, and ultimately central to how nurses structure the discipline of nursing" (p. 2). Silva, Sorrell, and Sorrell advocate for the inclusion of the inexplicable and the unknowable, which relate to the in-between and the beyond. The authors urge nurses to move past epistemological questions to ontological questions that deal with issues of reality, meaning, and being. They suggest questions such as "What does my perceptual sensibility to art reveal to me?" "How do I come to know the inexplicable and the unknowable?" and "What meaning do the inexplicable and unknowable have for me?" (p. 10). The authors maintain that through ontological study, a significant contribution to the foundation of nursing can be made. Such study would broaden and deepen our understanding of culture and support the ways in which culture influences our decisions.

Dialogue, Culture, and Knowing

According to Freire and Macedo (1995), dialogue is a way of knowing and "an indispensable component of the process of both learning and knowing" (p. 10). Theorizing about the experiences shared in dialogue is part and parcel of Freire's (2002) goal of learning and knowing. A curiosity about the object of knowledge must always be present. Dialogue is not an end; it is a way to better understanding. Dialogue, in this sense, can add immeasurably to an understanding of culture and culture's impact on the decisions that we make. The dialogue we engage in with patients and their families, for example, helps us shape our understanding of how healthcare decisions are made.

The following is a case study told by a doctorate of nursing practice student who had experience as a family nurse practitioner. This case study highlights how the dialectic can help in understanding a patient, their family, and their culture, as well as influence care and the outcomes of that care.

Case Study 2

A gentleman came to my practice for evaluation of an open wound to his right ankle. At first glance one could see that this man had very dark skin, and he spoke with a Jamaican accent. A vascular surgeon referred him to my practice. The surgeon called me prior to the patient's arrival and stated that this man had been referred to four or five doctors and yet continued to have an open wound. The surgeon stated he believed the man must practice some "Jamaican" religion where plant medicine was used because the man was applying tree "cooling" liquids to the open wound and this must be why it was not healing. The surgeon had used a narrow view when he evaluated this patient.

To help me understand this patient, I reflected back on my understanding of Jamaican culture that I had learned from a former patient and a colleague from that culture. For example, I had learned Jamaicans practice many religions and that their beliefs on health or health concepts are based on cold, gas/wind, heat, bile, blood imbalances, and germs. I knew this might be why my patient was using the "cooling" liquids on his wound. Jamaicans believe that an open wound can be the result of blood imbalances.

To learn more, I began to interview him and learned about his family, religious practices, environment, politics, social structure, genetics, and ethnohistory. From our conversation, I learned that the patient was of Jamaican descent with some Irish background, had lived in the United States for 18 years, was Roman Catholic, and had a wife and seven children. The patient's wife was currently living in Jamaica with four of the children; the three older children lived with their father.

The interview gave me time to learn about this person as well as why he came to the practice. He explained that he had had this wound for over a year, had been to his medical doctor many times, and was repeatedly referred to other specialists. He had no history of trauma or related medical illnesses such as diabetes. He stated that although he had health insurance, he only recently had taken to caring for the wound himself because he could no longer afford the time to see doctors whose treatments did not help.

A biopsy was performed in our office and 2 days later we received a diagnosis of invasive malignant melanoma. As soon as possible I spoke with the patient, who was relieved to get a diagnosis. I then ordered a full body CT scan and MRI of his brain. The tests uncovered multiple malignant nodes in his liver, abdomen, and chest. No metastasis was present in the brain. The patient would die of this disease within months to a year. After discussing this grave diagnosis with him, I referred him to oncology, where he agreed to have one round of interferon. He became very ill from the treatment and refused further chemotherapy. My patient then decided to return to Jamaica with his children to be with his wife and children and maintain a good quality of life with whatever time he had left. He also wanted to get his affairs in order.

Judging Other Cultures

Diversity, multiculturalism, and cultural competence are important concepts in nursing today (Jeffries, 2010; Leiniger & McFarland, 2006). The emphasis of these concepts should be on accepting and respecting cultural differences, making moral relativism an easy pitfall because there is little to guide professionals in making decisions. Diversity and multicultural populations are increasingly an important aspect of health care; thus, the ability to evaluate cultural practices is an important nursing skill worldwide. Multiculturalism in the international context asserts the claim that there are no common moral principles shared by all cultures. Postmodernism asserts a similar claim against all universal standards, both moral and nonmoral.

Important concepts related to culture are cultural imperialism, relativism, and imposition (Purnell & Paulanka, 2012). For this chapter only the perspectives of cultural imperialism and cultural imposition will be discussed. *Cultural imperialism*, often thought of as applying to the interactions of countries, also includes the imposition of the policies and practices of one organization onto another. Usually the transfer is from the dominant culture to disenfranchised or minority groups. *Cultural imposition* is the intrusive or disrespectful treatment of individuals and families by dominant culture practices. In health care, policies regarding visiting hours, food service, exclusion of families from plans of care, and informed consent can be seen as impositions. Purnell and Paulanka (2012) advise that nurses must be wary or prudent in expressing their own values.

This next case study, discussing the experience of another graduate nursing student, shows how universal standards of beauty vary and influence the kinds of healthcare decisions made surrounding, for example, obesity. Decisions about care from the perspective of the professional as well as from that of the individual, family, community, or population can differ based on cultural factors.

Case Study 3

I am reminded of a story I read a while ago of three young nurses who joined a medical mission to Mauritania, West Africa, where the culture was different from that of the U.S. nurses. When the nurses arrived in the assigned village, they saw that many girls were overweight. They agreed that their first challenge would be to teach weight control. As the days passed and the nurses treated patients in the local clinic, each thought about the problem they first encountered and how they might help the girls in the village deal with it.

One of the nurses thought she should distribute pamphlets to her patients. Few seemed interested in the materials, and in the evening she saw that some of the villagers used the pamphlets as kindling for their cooking fires. The second nurse thought that the overweight must be due to laziness. In the afternoon, she taught classes on exercise. She could not understand why her classes were not well-attended; every morning she ran alone. She also lectured about the value of keeping trim to anyone who would listen. She wondered how any man could find such overweight women attractive.

The third nurse, intrigued by the people she met in Mauritania, decided to find out as much as she could about their culture. She learned that obesity is considered to be quite attractive; it is actually valued in the community rather than a problem to be eradicated. Women learned that obesity makes them more appealing to a potential mate (Dayer-Barenson, 2011).

The moral is that just because a person's world view may differ from yours, that difference does not make it wrong.

What to Do When Making Decisions

To make an appropriate decision, we must first develop cultural awareness and sensitivity. Invest in knowing all that you can; be inquisitive, self-reflective, and aware of the various extant theories and models that can enhance your cultural sensitivity. The work of Leininger and McFarland (2006) and Jeffries (2010), for example, can offer insights and expand one's knowledge and knowing. Looking back on the patterns of knowing, see how you can develop acumen in each area. Science is probably the easiest to accomplish. As nurses and scholars we are comfortable with science. We have to keep abreast of developments and findings in nursing and other fields. Nurses know how to keep current in their specialization by reading journals, attending conferences, taking part in discussions, and so forth. Esthetics, the second way to know, can be decidedly fun, interesting, and even entertaining. Understanding and knowledge can be gleaned, for example, through film, fine art, crafts, dance, literature (fiction, nonfiction, and poetry), music and song, theater, museums of all types, and other cultural events. Literature is an especially rich source for gaining understanding and insight. For instance, female genital mutilation (FGM) is frequently in the news and it is generally laden with emotional response. A good place to start learning more about this topic is with the discussion by Nussbaum (1999). Nussbaum, a philosopher, presents a cogent, to-the-point argument with a lot of facts. To understand a piece of the unknowable, turn to Alice Walker's *Possessing the Secret of Joy* (1992). This novel is powerful and goes to the very core of FGM by making real the experience of one woman. Edwidge Danticat (1994) probes the issues further with an exploration of how FGM victimizes generations away from the actual cutting experience in her novel, *Breath, Eyes, Memory*.

As Carper (1978) suggests, personal knowing is the third and most difficult pattern to learn and inculcate into practice. Personal knowing is important in the actualization of an authentic relationship between two persons whose goal is to promote healing. It is learning and developing many characteristics of care-based ethics, which is rooted in receptivity, relatedness, and responsiveness (Noddings, 1984, 2002).

The ethics pattern of knowing has always been important to nurses. Theorists prescribe how nurses ought to act, although ethics may not be intrinsic to the theory but merely superimposed (Barnum, 1998). Like culture, ethics must be included in curricula so that nurses have the skills needed to recognize and work through situations that have ethics implications. To develop skill in identifying and resolving ethical issues, it is important to have the background knowledge to discuss problems and approaches to resolutions. The dialogue that Freire (2002) speaks of is very useful and helpful. It is important to understand that what is without dialogue and thus unexamined is not sufficient when encountering ethical discomfort and dilemmas.

The ontological in-between and beyond pattern of knowing is seen in phenomenologic and hermeneutic research and in the art, poetry, and narratives created by nurses (Silva et al., 1995). Again, study, read, have dialogues, engage with art, and create art by writing, painting, and so forth. This is important because it helps nurses to provide excellent patient care. The in-betweens and beyonds raise ontological questions about the world, about meaning, and about being. Information must not be blindly accepted; it must be critiqued and shared. Critical thinking is essential. All of the patterns of knowing require the dialogue of which Freire speaks. Without this dialogue, learning stands still and our world and our worldviews shrink.

Now that we have discussed patterns of knowing and how to develop those patterns, it must be acknowledged that breaking apart knowing in this way is a means to understand and gain access to the complexity of knowing. As Wilson (1998) eloquently stated, complexity with reductionism makes science whereas complexity without reductionism makes art. The patterns of knowing are not separate realms; they are extremely complex and interrelated. Understanding these patterns of knowing (and unknowing) and simultaneously linking them to ideas about culture supports a broader worldview when making decisions.

Culture, Critical Thinking, and Decision-Making

Culture must be considered in making many decisions, and critical thinking is essential. Collection of all pertinent data is imperative. Leininger (2002) asks the following questions: who benefits, who is harmed, what are the benefits, what are the harms? If there are harms associated with the practice or tradition, the decision becomes an ethical decision. In such a case, certain qualities are demanded of the decision maker. The decision maker must be able to recognize ethical issues and to think through the consequences of alternate resolutions. In the following case study, developed by a graduate student, issues related to legality, ethics, and harm versus tradition come into play, and she describes how she worked with her patient to mitigate harm.

Case Study 4

Obtaining consent for a procedure in the healthcare arena is second nature to practitioners. The practice in CT surgery is to explain the type of procedure, the sequence of events leading to the surgery, and the patient status during the immediate postoperative period. By the end of the speech, the patient seldom has a question, and the consent form is signed, dated, and witnessed.

At the eve of Yom Kippur this year, I had a different encounter. I admitted an Orthodox rabbi who presented with a 95 percent left main lesion and had active EKG changes and required intravenous anticoagulation. I proceeded with my speech to obtain permission for emergency surgery when I was told by the rabbi and his family that he would not be able to sign the consent, even with the understanding of the importance of immediate intervention. Surgery would have to be performed within 24 hours, but the holiday would not permit the use of a pen to give written consent. Time was of the essence, and religious beliefs dominated the moment.

I engaged in reflective practice by asking the following: How can I be instrumental in this unique situation? How can I expedite care while taking into consideration religious beliefs? Would I have to step out of legal boundaries? What are the consequences of inaction? I accepted the fact that permission was not going to be obtained in the routine format. My focus was to render care while respecting the religious restrictions.

I contacted patient services, who quickly educated me regarding the religious practice. In concert with legal services at my institution, a verbal consent was obtained with an event note documented and witnessed to expedite the procedure. The family showed relief and contentment when we announced that surgery would proceed as planned. The gratitude expressed by the rabbi was articulated months later via a letter to the chief of the department. I recall one sentence: "For this act of kindness and empathy, I felt healed prior to surgery and I thank you."

As shown in this case study, the decision maker must have the self-confidence to seek out different points of view and then decide what is right at a given time and place in terms of a particular set of relationships and combination of circumstances. Jeffries (2010) refers to a "perceived confidence" when she writes about transcultural self-efficacy. Transcultural self-efficacy is defined as the nurse's "confidence for performing or learning general transcultural nursing skills among culturally different clients" (p. 46), and it is part of Jeffries's Cultural Competence and Confidence Model, a tool that can be used when making decisions. We must learn all we can about the situation in order to be able to reach the best decision. Finally, the decision maker must be willing to make decisions when all that needs to be known cannot be known and the questions that press for answers have no established and incontrovertible solution.

Summary

We must remember that culture is not static; culture is ever changing. North American culture is very different at the beginning of the twenty-first century than it was 50 or 100 years ago, or than it was at its founding. A culture is made up of a plurality of people who have different relationships of power to one another. Some of these relationships are nurturing and sustaining; others may be pathological and detrimental to human flourishing. Nurses must recognize that there are universal principles to protect human flourishing and dignity and we must learn to make decisions that do so.

References

Andrews, M. M., & Boyle, J. S. (2012). *Transcultural concepts in nursing care* (6th ed.). New York: Lippincott, Williams & Wilkins.

Bach, P. B, Pham, H. H., Schrag, D., Tate, R. C., & Hargraves, J. L. (2004). Primary care physicians who treat blacks and whites. *New England Journal of Medicine, 351*, 575–584.

Barnum, B. S. (1998). *Nursing theory: Analysis, application, evaluation*. New York: Lippincott, Williams & Wilkins.

Beauchamp, T., & Childress, J. (2009). *Principles of biomedical ethics* (6th ed.). New York: Oxford University Press.

Blackburn, S. (1996). *Oxford dictionary of philosophy*. New York: Oxford University Press.

Bloche, M. (2004). Health care disparities: Science, politics, and race. *New England Journal of Medicine, 350*, 1568–1570.

Cameron-Traub, E. (2002). Western ethical, moral, and legal dimensions within the culture care theory. In M. M. Leininger & M. R. McFarland (Eds.), *Transcultural nursing: Concepts, theories, research, and practice* (3rd ed., pp. 169–177). New York: McGraw-Hill.

Carper, B. (1978). Fundamental patterns of knowing in nursing. *Advances in Nursing Science, 1*(1), 13–23.

Chernow, B. A., & Vallasi, G. A. (1993). *The Columbia encyclopedia* (5th ed.). New York: Columbia University Press.

Chinn, P. L., & Kramer, M. K. (1991). *Theory and nursing: A systematic approach* (3rd ed.). St. Louis, MO: Mosby-Yearbook.

Danticat, E. (1994). *Breath, eyes, memory*. New York: Vintage Books.

Dayer-Berenson, L. (2011). *Cultural competencies for nurses: Impact on health and illness*. Sudbury, MA: Jones & Bartlett.

Dickson, P. R. (1994). The shared values that make an organizational culture. In *Marketing management*. New York: Dryden Press.

Ebby, R. A., Hartley, P. L., Hodges, J., Hoffpauir, R., Newbanks, S., & Kelley, J. H. (2013). Moral integrity and moral courage: Can you teach it? *Journal of Nursing Education, 52*(4), 229–233.

Eckroth-Bucher, M. (2010). Self-awareness: A review and analysis of a basic nursing concept. *Advances in Nursing Science, 33*(4), 297–309.

Freire, P. (2002). *Pedagogy of the oppressed* (trans. M. B. Ramos). New York: Continuum Publishing Company.

Freire, P., & Macedo, D. (1995). A dialogue: Culture, language, and race. *Harvard Educational Review, 65*(3), 379.

Haiman, C. A., Stram, D. O., Wilkins, L. R., Pike, M. C., Kolonel, L. N., Henderson, B. E., & Le Marchand, L. (2006). Ethnic and racial differences in smoking-related risk of lung cancer. *New England Journal of Medicine*, 354(4), 333–342.

Jeffries, M. R. (2010). *Teaching cultural competence in nursing and health care* (2nd ed.). New York: Springer Publishing Company.

Johnson, J. L. (1994). A dialectical examination of nursing art. *Advances in Nursing Science, 17*(1), 1–14.

Ketefian, S., & Redman, R. W. (1977). Nursing science in the global community. *Image: Journal of Nursing Scholarship*, 29, 11–15.

Kramer, M. (1974). *Reality shock: Why nurses leave nursing*. St. Louis, MO: C.V. Mosby.

Kramer, M., & Schmalenberg, C. (1977). *Path to biculturalism*. Wakefield, MA: Contemporary Publishing Company.

Leininger, M. M. (2002). Part I: The theory of culture care and ethnonursing research method. In M. M. Leininger & M. R. McFarland (Eds.), *Transcultural nursing: Concepts, theories, research, and practice* (3rd ed., pp. 71–116). New York: McGraw-Hill.

Leininger, M. M., & McFarland, M. R. (2006). *Culture care diversity and universality: A worldwide nursing theory* (2nd ed.). Sudbury, MA: Jones & Bartlett.

Macklin, R. (1999). *Against relativism: Cultural diversity and the search for ethical universals in medicine*. New York: Oxford University Press.

Munhall, P. (1993). "Unknowing": Toward another pattern of knowing in nursing. *Nursing Outlook*, 41, 125–128.

National Research Council and Institute of Medicine. (2013). *United States health in international perspective: Shorter lives, poorer health*. S. H. Woolf & L. Aron (Eds.). Washington, DC: National Academies Press.

Noddings, N. (1984). *Caring: A feminine approach to ethics and moral education*. Berkeley, CA: University of California Press.

Noddings, N. (2002). *Starting at home: Caring and social policy*. Berkeley, CA: University of California Press.

Nussbaum, M.C. (1999). *Sex and social justice*. New York: Oxford University Press.

Porter-O'Grady, T., & Malloch, K. (2011). *Quantum leadership: Advancing innovation, transforming health care* (3rd ed). Sudbury, MA: Jones & Bartlett.

Purnell, L. D., & Paulanka, B. J. (Eds.). (2012). *Transcultural health care: A culturally competent approach* (4th ed.). Philadelphia: F.A. Davis.

Rogers, M. E. (1988). Nursing science and art: A perspective. *Nursing Science Quarterly, 1*, 99–102.

Silva, M. C., Sorrell, J. M., & Sorrell, C. D. (1995). From Carper's patterns of knowing to ways of being: An ontological philosophical shift in nursing. *Advances in Nursing Science, 18*(1), 1–13.

Smedley, B. D., Stith, A. Y., & Nelson, A. R. (2003). *Unequal treatment: Confronting racial and ethnic disparities in health care*. Washington, DC: National Academies Press.

Steinbrook, R. (2004). Disparities in health care: From politics to policy. *New England Journal of Medicine, 350*, 1486–1488.

Walker, A. (1992). *Possessing the secret of joy*. New York: Harcourt Brace Jovanovich.

Wilson, E. O. (1998). *Consilience: The unity of knowledge*. New York: Alfred A. Knopf.

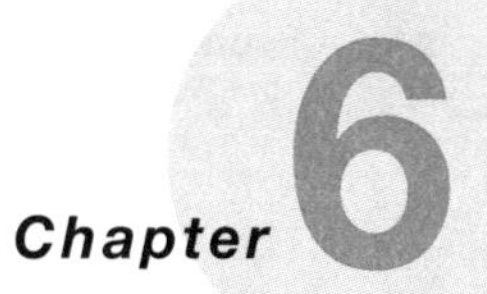

Chapter 6

Family and Decision-Making

Susan Salmond

Health is created and lived by people within the settings of their everyday life where they learn, work, play, and love (World Health Organization, 1986). Families are a key component of this setting and are considered one of the most important influencing factors on one's health. Families are primary sources of support and are generally the first place a person turns when challenged with serious illness. Family support may take the form of expressions of caring and love, practical assistance with activities of daily living, instrumental assistance, support of role change, help with regimen adherence, and support with decision-making (Eel, 1996; Feinberg, Reinhard, Houser, & Choula, 2011; Friedman, 2002). As of 2009, there were approximately 65.7 million informal family caregivers providing care to someone who was ill, disabled, or aged in the United States (National Alliance for Caregiving & AARP, 2009). This converts to an economic value of approximately $450 billion in unpaid contributions (Feinberg et al., 2011).

When disease or injury disrupts a person's health, there is a ripple effect that extends outward from the person to family and friends and into the community itself (Salmond & Spears, 2002). This ripple can be experienced as a gentle movement or more like a tidal wave as families are called upon to make important life and lifestyle decisions in partnership with or on behalf of the patient, to serve as caregivers, and to advocate within the stormy seas of the healthcare system for their ill loved one. The explicit recognition of the critical role that families play in caregiving and maximizing health is central to care grounded in a family-centered paradigm. Despite widespread endorsement of the notion of patient- and family-centered care, it continues to be insufficiently implemented in clinical practice (Abraham & Moretz, 2012; Institute of Medicine, 2001; Zuo et al., 2012).

What Is Patient (Person)- and Family-Centered Care (PFCC)?

In the landmark report, *Crossing the Quality Chasm* (2001), the Institute of Medicine (IOM) defined patient-centered care as the provision of care that is "respectful of and responsive to individual patient preferences, needs and values and ensuring that patient values guide all clinical decisions" (p. 40). Feinberg (2012) suggests using the terminology *person-centered care* because it is more reflective of the whole person. She contends that *patient* is a term grounded in the medical context with a focus on "health care providers, specific diseases, episodes of care, and office visits to clinicians" (p. 2). In contrast, person-centered care goes beyond this paradigm and "emphasizes continuity of care, support and quality of life" (Feinberg, 2012 p. 2). Family-centered care amplifies person-centered care by acknowledging and reinforcing the vital role of family caregivers not only in the "planning and delivery of supportive services," but also in acknowledging "family needs and preferences and integrate[ing] family caregivers as partners in care" (Feinberg, Reinhard, Houser, & Choula, 2011, p. 10).

PFCC places the patient and family, the experts regarding that person's illness experience, at the center of the care team in a meaningful and respectful partnership approach to healthcare planning, delivery, evaluation, and decision-making (Christensen, 2007; Feinberg, 2011; Institute for Patient- and Family-Centered Care [IPFCC], n.d. a,b; Zuo et al., 2012). The IOM highlights four key tenets of PFCC: respect and dignity, information sharing, participation, and collaboration. These key tenets are further defined in **Table 6-1**. Berwick (2009) builds on these tenets and defines patient-centered care as "the experience (to the extent the informed, individual patient desires it) of transparency, individualization, recognition, respect, dignity, and choice in all matters, without exception, related to one's person, circumstances, and relationships in health care." He further contends that "in most circumstances, people would, and should be able to expand this approach to include the experience of family and loved ones of their choosing—PFCC" (pp. 560–561).

PFCC is not one intervention but multiple interventions and interactions that support a philosophical approach to care that recognizes the needs of patients and patients' family members, acknowledging the important role those family members play during a patient's illness (Henneman & Cardin, 2002). It is a complete turn away from the paternalistic model in which nurses and doctors have all the answers and dictate to patients. In PFCC, the patient and family are valued as key members of the team. They provide guidance on what is actually happening, on what medication works best for them, on what a caregiver has forgotten to do or has done incorrectly, and on what treatment option they feel would be best based on their life context and values. In essence, the patient and family are the key to safety and quality,

PFCC has long been acknowledged as the model of care in pediatric and community nursing. With the growing evidence that engaging patients and families as partners leads to improved health outcomes, satisfaction, and quality care, the call for PFCC in all health settings and with all populations has intensified (Balik, Conway, Zipperer, & Watson, 2011; James, 2013; Institute of Medicine, 2001). Leading the move for PFCC from a "nice" approach to a necessary approach is the Centers for Medicare and Medicaid Services (CMS), in that they have made PFCC a performance requirement equal to those in clinical quality, safety, and finance. Future reimbursement (value-based incentive payments)

Table 6-1

Key Tenets of PFCC	
Dignity and respect	The healthcare provider listens to patients and families. Their ideas and choices are respected. Their knowledge, values, beliefs, and cultural backgrounds are understood and appreciated and used to improve care planning and delivery.
Information sharing	The healthcare provider communicates and shares complete and unbiased information with patients and families in useful ways. Patients and families receive timely, complete, and accurate details so they can take part in care and decision-making.
Involvement	Patients and families are encouraged and supported to participate in care and decision-making at the level they choose.
Collaboration	Patients and family members are invited to work together with healthcare staff to develop and evaluate policies and programs.

Source: Johnson, Abraham, Conway, Simmons, Edgman-Levitan, Sodomka, Schlucter, & Ford (2008). *Partnering with patients and families to design a patient- and family-centered health care system.* Reprinted with permission from the Institute for Patient- and Family-Centered Care: www.ipfcc.org.

will be based in part on patient experience. The measure of the success of PFCC is complex, but clearly a central domain will be measures of satisfaction with care. The incentive for change is quite clear. It is a priority for nurses, other healthcare providers, and organizational systems themselves to put patients and families at the center of care, not only in name but in practice.

Moving to a PFCC approach in one's individual care as well as across a unit and organization is a major paradigm shift. Nurses and other care providers need to examine their underlying beliefs about control in healthcare decision-making and participation of the family as an equal on the team. PFCC changes the approach to how care is delivered and moves processes from a provider- or organization-centric position to one with greater flexibility for responding to patient and family needs. Berwick (2009) contends that an organization that truly adopts PFCC would be radically and uncomfortably different from most today. Some of the changes that come with this model include few restrictions on visiting hours, patients and families participating in rounds and change of shift reports, medical records belonging to patients, councils of patients and families helping to guide design of healthcare processes and services, and patients and families being actively involved in decision-making about their care—what it will be and how it will be delivered.

Who Is the Family?

Who makes up a family is not decided by the caregiver. Family is whomever the patient chooses to call family (Balik et al., 2011). This broad definition of family is consistent with current thinking on relationships within contemporary society. No longer is the traditional nuclear family the mainstay of family structure in the United States. In fact, "fully half of all families do not meet the definition of nuclear family" (American Academy of Pediatrics [AAP], 2013, para 1). The structure of the family varies and may include:

> ...nuclear, stepfamily, single-parent family, families headed by two unmarried partners—either of the opposite sex or the same sex, households that include one or more family members from a generation, adoptive families, foster families, and families where children are raised by their grandparents or other relatives. One is not better than the other. Each has its distinctive advantages and challenges. (AAP, 2013, para 1)

Giving people the opportunity to decide who family is allows them to include birth families and families of choice. Nurses who have a narrower definition of family, such as a traditional nuclear family, may fail to engage the appropriate individuals, causing significant anxiety, disappointment, anger, resentment, and family and patient stress as well as health deficits for both the patient and the family. How to avoid this? All nurses should start by looking inward and self-reflecting on their own thoughts and feelings regarding family. Consider your thoughts on heterosexuality and homosexuality, nuclear and extended families, married and unmarried partners, and fictive kin as family, and your thoughts surrounding expected role patterns in families. Once aware of your own beliefs and values, it is possible to turn outward and examine whether these beliefs support or hinder embracing the family as a care partner. Responding therapeutically to persons from all family types is facilitated when guided by the understanding that kinship and its connections and close ties to others are part of health and well-being, and these "kin" are likely to play an essential role in helping a loved one cope with and adjust to illness or injury.

Knowing that family is defined by the perception of the patient and that there are many different types of families, avoid making automatic assumptions; instead, ask, "Who do you consider family?" or "Who do you want to be involved in your care?" or "What family would you like involved in your care?" Don't worry how your question sounds; the question is likely to elicit the necessary contextual information for understanding what constitutes family to this person. When the healthcare team engages the patient and the relevant family focusing on both the immediate and longer term health concerns, empowerment occurs, a "healthy family" concept is promoted, and better patient and family outcomes are achieved (Burchard, 2005).

The Impact of Illness on the Family

Fear and anxiety are common emotions for family members as they cope with the uncertainty of illness and their inability to balance change and maintain stability in an environment that is unfamiliar and frequently frightening. Their loved one may be at risk for dying or suffering ongoing deficits, and together with unplanned changing family roles, a precarious family situation evolves (Mitchell, Courney, & Coyer, 2003). Some families may appear overwhelmed with emotions and others may seem confident, knowledgeable, and articulate, but they are all dealing with horror and fright and a depth of emotion and turmoil (Taylor, 2006).

When a loved one is hospitalized (and often when they attend clinics and other appointments) they are asked to hand over care to strangers and there are concerns regarding competency and consistency of care. Within what is often an impersonal hospital environment, establishing a respectful relationship between the family and the nurse is crucial. Facilitating open and honest communication and responding to common family concerns are critical components to establishing this relationship. Leske's (1991) systematic review of family needs during acute illness identified three common needs that exist: the need for assurance, the need for proximity, and the need for information. Consciously or unconsciously, nurses control the level of family stress and participation by controlling behavior that impacts these three areas (Corlett & Twycross, 2006).

In a PFCC model, the nurse gives assurance through respect, involvement, and collaboration—listening to what the person and family say, gaining an understanding of their illness experience, and explicitly encouraging them to be active partners on the team. Assurance is also associated with perceptions of nursing competence. Conveying and demonstrating competence about your ability to provide effective care will assure the family; its absence is one of the strongest predictors of family dissatisfaction (Hunziker et al., 2012).

The need for proximity is met by involvement and being flexible with policies that limit family presence. In a PFCC model, family members (as determined by the patient) are considered key caregivers, participate in healthcare visits, assist with care provision, are part of the discussion during rounds, and often remain present during invasive procedures. Being proactive to promote family visitation and involvement in the patient's care allows the family to remain emotionally close and to give support to the patient and guidance to the healthcare team. Assigning a nurse contact for the family is an excellent strategy for communication so that the family knows to whom they can direct their questions and be provided information on patient status.

The last need, information sharing, is key to the advocacy role that families take on in PFCC. Nurses are gatekeepers to patients and families receiving complete and unbiased information. Providing information diminishes some of the anxiety and uncertainty experienced, and reciprocal information sharing is part of establishing rapport (Espezel & Canam, 2003). The nurse should explain presenting symptoms and treatments in a meaningful way so that patterns become recognizable and treatment makes sense in light of the symptoms. The present situation should be compared to the patient's prior condition or previous episodes so that patients and families can recognize patterns. Information giving must accommodate the family's expected high anxiety: Avoid professional jargon, plan for repetition of information, ask the family what they understand about the situation, use teach-back approaches, provide information based on their understanding and any evident gaps, give opportunities to ask questions and solicit more information, and give emotional support. Supplement conversations or teaching sessions with videotapes or DVDs, information booklets, or care conferences.

The nurse plays another major role in helping the family to integrate the different information being received from an array of providers. Families verbalize frustration with inconsistent and conflicting information as well as with receiving only isolated bits of information at a time. The nurse can play a significant role as coordinator for information coming in "system bytes" as one specialist sees a patient and provides information on the kidneys and another specialist sees the patient and provides information on the pulmonary status. Often families interpret specialist information generally. In other words, if the nephrologist says that the kidneys are doing fine, then the family may interpret this as the patient is improving, even if their neurological condition is deteriorating. Help the family to see the "big picture" by interpreting the information in light of the patient's overall condition. Do not take away hope, but assist the family in understanding the whole.

Another value of the family-centered approach to care is the potential preventative role that the model can take. Families are at risk of adverse outcomes as a result of critical or prolonged chronic illness of a loved one. Family caregivers' own health will be tested by the physical and emotional work of caring (Radcliffe, Adeshokan, Thompson, & Bakowski, 2012). Anxiety, depression, somatization, and symptoms of posttraumatic stress disorder have been found to occur in these families (Cook, 2001). Recognizing the vulnerability of family caregivers and reducing caregiver strain is an important component of PFCC (Feinberg, 2012). Attending to family needs as part of the care model can help the family to cope with the situation as well as find resources and strategies to support their own needs.

The Family Role in the Illness Experience

Families influence and are influenced by the health of their members. They assume important roles in health promotion and risk reduction, advocate and coordinate care for the individual experiencing acute and chronic illness, and are instrumental as sources of either stress or support as individuals cope with illness. Family members act as buffers for patient anxiety and serve as valuable resources for care, typically acting as the main source of help for family members with functional limitations (Cannon, 2011; Feinberg, 2012). The family can be an ally and a source of information about the patient's condition and can help the healthcare team to be more effective in planning and delivering care for their loved one (Katz, 2012). Families have detailed information about their family member that can help not only to diagnosis a problem, but also to detect subtle changes signifying improvement or deterioration in the patient (Frazee, 2011). They know the person and can provide information on how that person is responding to care. They know how the person looks today and how the person looked 12 days ago—something that the care provider does not know. Their knowledge is a crucial part of assuring safety and quality.

> A consistent family caregiver—across all transitions of care and care settings—will recognize his or her loved one as a whole person, not focusing exclusively on a specific disease, disorder or episode of hospital care. They can become the patient's "eyes and ears," recognizing changes in symptoms and function that may necessitate different care or supports. (Feinberg, 2011, p. 2)

Typically health care is delivered in episodes. The acute care nurse focuses on the acute physiologic instability, the home care nurse on helping the patient manage once home, and the ambulatory care nurse on the purpose of the visit. There is a disconnect with this narrow focus and the context of what is happening to the patient, why it happened, and what needs to be done to prepare the patient and family to effectively self-manage and to coordinate transitions of care. PFCC sees the nurse and other healthcare providers as responsible for clinical management and the patient and family as responsible for self-management. With meaningful engagement and partnership, the focus is not on doing things for and to the patient but on directly involving patients and families in the continuum of care and including them in defining the problems, deciding on best options, and building the knowledge and skills needed for self-management. In this way both the clinical management and self-management are addressed, thereby facilitating transitions of care that are seamless.

Healthcare providers underestimate the extent to which families want to be involved; only a minority of patients and family achieve the desired level of involvement (Hack, Degner, Watson, & Sinha, 2005; Osborn et al., 2012; Stricker et al., 2009). Hanson and Barach (2012) remind us that managing a patient "in a reliable and safe manner requires patients and nurses to partner together to achieve optimal outcomes" (p. 74).

Family Management Styles: One Size Does Not Fit All

One must begin with the premise that there is no "one size fits all" approach for family interaction. Each family presents with their unique family structure, caring styles, family strengths and challenges, and roles they play in the trajectory of the disease. There will be a negotiation process in which it will be determined what the family participation will consist of and what roles the family will have in sharing care of their sick relative and in the decision-making process.

Families will have different preferences for information and for involvement in decision-making and may range from avoidance to active engagement. Benbassat, Pilpel, and Tidhar (1998) identified factors associated with preference for a passive role, including minority status, less education, being elderly, and more severe illness. They concluded that desire for information was more universal, but there was greater variability with preferred degrees of participation in decision-making. Although many accounts suggest that some patients prefer to leave their healthcare decisions to their healthcare providers, Long's (2013) study of low-income Californian residents found when these residents were given the option to be clearly informed about the treatment choices that were medically appropriate for them (rather than simply making the decision), 81 percent opted to participate in shared decision-making. The nurse plays a significant role in assuring that patents and families receive understandable information in order to participate in decision-making.

The level of involvement desired needs to be assessed. Do they want in-depth information or just enough to understand? Do they want to be involved in collaborating on decisions related to treatment or delegate decision-making to healthcare providers? Recognize that these preferences are not constant but are likely to change as the condition of the patient changes, families become more experienced with illness management, and other life circumstances intervene. An awareness of preferences will allow for tailoring of information as well as the level of decision-making.

Sobo (2004) emphasizes that preference for information may not be the same as preference for involvement in treatment decisions. Some families may engage in information exchange without decision-making whereas others may want to engage in both. In order to tailor the intervention to be appropriate to the patient and family, the nurse should ask the patient and/or family two clarifying questions about information and decision-making preferences.

1. When possible, what level of information would you prefer to receive?
   - The simplest information possible
   - More than the simplest information, but keep it on everyday terms
   - In-depth information that I can help you understand
   - As much in-depth and detailed information as can be provided

2. When possible, and with the appropriate information support provided to you, what decision-making role do you (patient and/or family) want to assume?
    - Leave all decisions about care to the care team.
    - Have the care team make decisions about care with serious consideration of our views.
    - Share in making the decisions about care with the care team.
    - Make all decisions about care with serious consideration of the care team's advice.
    - Make all decisions about care.

With the answers to these two critical questions, the nurse can ask: Compared to what is desired, is the current level of information giving and decision-making on target? This assessment needs to be an ongoing process because it is likely that the family members' interest in participation will change based on the disease trajectory and whether they experience care that truly values their partnership.

Intentional Nursing Actions to Support PFCC

The single most important recommendation for involving patients and families is to believe that participation is important. Examining one's attitudes is a preliminary step for each nurse. Consider your beliefs in regards to the following questions taken from the Institute for Patient- and Family-Centered Care's resource, *Advancing the Practice of Patient- and Family-Centered Care* (IPFCC, n.d. a,b) within the hospital and primary care and ambulatory settings. When examining your clinical interaction with each patient and family, consider the following: Do I view patients and families as essential members of the healthcare team? Do I believe that patients and family members bring unique perspectives and expertise to the clinical relationship? Do I encourage families to speak freely? Do I listen respectfully to the opinions of patients and family members? Do I encourage patients and family members to participate in decision-making about their care? Do I encourage patients and family members to be active partners in assuring the safety and quality of their own care? This can be elevated to the unit level by asking yourself whether you consistently let colleagues know that you value the insights of patients and families and using these same questions to determine the majority view of providers on the unit.

Although nurses should not be solely responsible for advancing PFCC, it is at the point of care where partnership practices come alive (Abraham & Moretz, 2012). Nurses who consistently partner with patients and families in daily care can become the champions or role models and mentors for others.

Nursing Care Promotes Dignity and Respect

Berwick (2009) reminds us that caregivers are guests in the patient's life and our interactions are opportunities to learn more together to achieve better health outcomes. Respectful interactions that maintain the patient's and family's dignity are the framework from which all other care emerges. Nursing care is responsive to both the patient and family, addressing their needs for physical comfort; emotional, informational, cultural, and spiritual support; and learning (Balick et al., 2011).

Ask the patient who is part of his or her family and then proactively reach out to the family and share the value of caring in partnership. Engage the family by asking them to tell you about the patient and themselves (the family). This begins to build a connection and provides valuable insight into the family and illness context. Learn more about the illness experience.

Information Giving and Sharing

Information is critical to advocacy and decision-making, yet many families indicate that healthcare providers do not provide the needed information. This is especially true when it comes to information addressing the social, lifestyle, and financial concerns associated with the illness experience—all important aspects of self-management (Hawkins et al., 2008). Sometimes needed information is given; however, it is not perceived as valuable because it is not provided in a meaningful way to the patient and family. In fact, it is often reported as confusing and unintelligible and surely does not provide the knowledge needed for active decision-making. All information and educational materials should not only be linguistically appropriate, but also written in a plain language style that avoids (or at least explains) medical jargon.

Nurses need to be approachable and proactive in their approach to forming patient and family relationships and in providing information. Families often do not know how to ask for what is needed or even what to ask for. Some families have had negative experiences when requesting information and hesitate to speak up, often take the path of least resistance, and don't articulate their needs. Recognize that it takes both energy and courage to speak up and request information or demand specific care interventions. Families fear alienating themselves from the very people that they rely on (Taylor, 2006).

Creating a culture that gives permission for families to disagree with or question the care received requires the nurses to adopt a family-centered approach. Respect for the family and interventions that are family inclusive are needed. In care planning, consider: How can I support the family today? What are they saying? What are they feeling? What are they not saying? As you interact with the family and have an opportunity to talk with them, focus on what the experience must be like for the patient. Ask them: What is it like when . . . ? What do you find hardest? What are some of the most frustrating aspects of this hospitalization/this illness/this regimen? What would you like to see done differently? What information do you need to help you manage the situation (Taylor, 2006)? What information is needed to support self-management and caregiving? What do the patient and family need to do at home in order to manage the disease and the regimen? Valuable resources for caregiving can be found at sites such as Next Step in Care (www.nextstepincare.org).

Involving the family in healthcare team rounds and walking report (handoff) are excellent opportunities for information sharing. Clarify the purpose of the rounds or report and welcome the family involvement. Remind the family that the nurses and doctors are the medical experts, but the patient and family are the experts on the patient and the self-management of the disease. While doing walking rounds, tell the patient and family that you are going to summarize the patient's story from that shift and that they should feel free to speak up if anything is omitted or is inaccurate. Ask whether there are questions, and whether the care delivered during the shift could have been provided in a manner that was more helpful and meaningful. This exchange of information allows for adapting care to best fit the needs of the patient and family.

Involvement and Shared Decision-Making

There are multiple ways in which nurses can proactively invite patients and families to participate as a partner in the care relationship. Use "we" language (e.g., We will be working together to provide care that meets your expectations). Discuss with the patient and family what they should expect from the nursing staff as well as the rest of the team and teach them to speak up with a reminder when that care is not delivered. Use "teach-back" methods as part of teaching encounters to actively engage the patient and family and identify areas of misunderstanding and confusion (Ahmann & Dokken, 2012). Remind patients and families that "questions are the answers" (Agency for Healthcare Research and Quality, n.d.) so they appreciate that the team truly wants their participation. Provide the patient and family with a journal so they can track concerns and questions, which can be discussed at set times. Having patients and family actively participate in rounds and change of shift report provides input into creation and evaluation of the plan of care.

Family decision-making can be a highly stressful process. Individual family members often wonder: Do I have the information I need? How do I decide when there is no clear-cut answer? What if I make the wrong decision? These are common concerns, especially among families of acutely ill patients where high uncertainty and often risky decisions are made under conditions of high emotional stress and time constraints (Pierce & Hicks, 2001). A well-informed person who is connected to their care providers is best prepared to participate in shared decision-making.

Shared decision-making (SDM) is a process of "active participation from the patient, family member and the professional to work together as partners in the decision-making process" (D'Aloja et al., 2010). In SDM, all parties discuss treatment options (as opposed to a single option based on provider preference), risks/benefits of the different options, and patient and family preferences and values that are relevant to reaching a joint decision. SDM can be used to decide on a patient's daily treatment and nursing care plan while in the hospital or used to decide on a treatment course for the management of a disease or condition. It is especially valuable in those situations where there are "preference-sensitive" conditions or treatment options.

SDM requires that a practitioner seek not only to understand each patient's needs and develop reasonable alternatives to meet those needs, but also to present the alternatives in a way that enables patients to choose one they prefer. Makoul and Clayman (2006) identified the essential elements of SDM to include:

- Definition/explanation of the problem
- Presentation of evidence-based treatment options
- Discussion of pros and cons of treatment options on prognosis and quality of life
- Discussion of patient and family values/preferences
- Discussion of patient and family strengths, abilities, and self-efficacy
- Discussion of nurse/physician recommendations
- Checking and clarifying patient and family understanding
- Making or explicitly deferring the decision
- Arranging follow-up

The SDM process may be facilitated with the use of decision aids (DA). Whether leaflets, books, DVDs, Web sites, or other interactive media, DAs give information about the risks and benefits of various treatment options and help the patient and family make choices that most reflect their personal values (James, 2013). They are not intended to replace discussion with healthcare providers, but rather to support an interaction in which the healthcare provider and the patient and family members exchange information and clarify values in order to reach a decision regarding medical treatment (Sheehan & Sherman, 2011). Sheehan and Sherman's systematic review led to the conclusion that one of the most consistent benefits of DAs was improved knowledge of options and outcomes. The benefits were not as strong with simpler aids as compared to detailed DAs and computer-interactive DAs. The more detailed and computer-interactive DAs supported values clarification and reduced decisional conflict. The Ottawa Personal Decision Guide is an example of a general DA that can be used to guide health decision-making. This is available at http://decisionaid.ohri.ca/docs/das/OPDG.pdf. The Ottawa site, as well as other sites such as eMedicine Health, provide condition-specific DAs that can be used in SDM. One such example is Low Back Pain: Should I Have an MRI, which can be found at: www.emedicinehealth.com/script/main/art.asp?articlekey=127380&ref=129885.

Option grids are another option for SDM; they are short tools for comparing health treatment options. They are easy to read and provide a framework for discussing decisions regarding treatment options. They allow for comparison of the options and answer common questions about the options. Examples of option grids can be found at www.optiongrid.org.

Collaboration

Collaboration of patients and families at the organizational level is needed to design processes of care, policies, and programs that are indeed patient and family friendly and support the nurses' practice in providing patient- and family-centered care. The structures and processes that are of priority importance include the admission assessment, bedside rounds, family meetings, communication strategies, discharge planning, and patient and family education (Walton, 2011). Patient and family advisors, who are former clients of the organization, assume roles in an advisory capacity (Warren, 2012). Capturing this experiential knowledge to move towards meaningful structural change is an organizational strategy to embed PFCC in the culture of the organization. A valuable site to support this process includes the Institute for Healthcare Improvement (www.ihi.org).

Case Study

The following case study demonstrates PFCC in action. The case study represents the first 4 days of an ICU experience.

Lisa S., age 33, was a direct admission via ambulance into the intensive care unit with a diagnosis of generalized status epilepticus.

She had been in a neighboring hospital for 2 days and was being transferred to a neurointensive care unit because her condition was not resolving. Lisa was accompanied by her long-term partner, and at the time of transfer into the ICU unit Marie was asked if she would be more comfortable remaining with Lisa or staying in the waiting area where someone would routinely bring information until that time when Lisa was assessed and stabilized. Marie requested to remain with Lisa. In this initial period, Lisa was intubated and placed on mechanical ventilation, an arterial line was placed, and continuous EEG monitoring initiated and ultimately mediated to achieve a propofol-induced coma. Coming into the room, a nurse let the team know that Marie would be observing and she was Lisa's life partner. While Lisa was being stabilized, a nurse and subsequently a chaplain stayed with Marie and explained to her what was happening, describing the equipment, the purpose of it, and why it was thought necessary in this emergency situation. While treating Lisa, the neurologist asked about Lisa's epilepsy history, the current episode, and medication history. After propofol administration, the visible rhythmic jerking ceased, which had a calming effect on Marie. The nurse and neurologist remained with Marie to explain the treatment and answer questions. Marie knew prior to coming to this hospital that the treatment was to be the propofol-induced coma. When questioned about what she expected would happen, she believed Lisa would be responsive shortly. She was then provided information that Lisa continued to have nonconvulsive seizures, so the medication would be continued and additional treatment initiated. The 24-hour EEG was explained.

The nurse explained to Marie that she could stay with Lisa as desired and gave her a phone number for calling in for updates when she chose to go home. Marie indicated that she wanted to stay and shared that she monitored much of Lisa's medical care. Marie and the nurse discussed Marie's role as a partner on the team and that together they would work towards the best achievable outcomes. Marie's interest in receiving information and participating in decision-making was assessed, and it was determined that Marie had in-depth knowledge of the disease and treatment and that she wanted the same in-depth information to understand what was happening to Lisa. Clearly Marie wanted to continue her decision-making role regarding Lisa's care. Marie was reassured by this relationship and the knowledge of the nurses in providing care. Over the next few days, the nurses engaged Marie in conversation and began to learn about Lisa as a person. Some of this information was converted into the plan of care. For instance, she had a love for gospel music, so Marie's iPod was hooked to speakers and gospel music was played. The nurses engaged Marie in a discussion of possible complications associated with immobility, and together they developed a plan of care that included Marie doing passive range of motion exercises with Lisa multiple times per day. Marie also assisted with basic care activities, assisting with bathing, turning, and providing skin care. The nurses consistently interacted with Marie, supporting her and inquiring about her emotional well-being and encouraging dialogue about her fears and concerns. She was given a journal for recording her observations and questions. When asked about her greatest fears, she verbalized fear of cognitive deficits as well as concern that Lisa would lose her job because she did not have much sick time. Marie herself was a school teacher and because it was a summer month, she had greater flexibility than at other times.

Interdisciplinary rounds were held at 9 each morning and Marie was an active participant. Marie was the first to bring up the need to get Lisa out of bed, despite her coma status; she had concerns about the Foley as a precautionary measure to avoiding urinary tract infection, and it was subsequently removed. She was also the first to report on altered stool activity, which subsequently was diagnosed as *C. difficile*. Subsequently she held everyone entering the room accountable for washing their hands. She had many questions regarding anticipated recovery and likelihood of subsequent clinical seizure activity. All questions were answered, and in many cases pathophysiologic explanations were given because Marie wanted to understand what was happening. Assurance, proximity, and information needs were continually met. She was treated with respect and dignity, and was actively involved while care was being delivered in a respectful way to her partner Lisa.

References

Abraham, M., & Moretz, J. G. (2012). Implementing patient- and family-centered care: Part 1—Understanding the challenges. *Pediatric Nursing*, 38(1), 44–47.

Agency for Healthcare Research and Quality (n.d.). *Questions are the answer.* Retrieved from http://www.ahrq.gov/legacy/questions/index.html

Ahmann, E., & Dokken, D. (2012). Strategies for encouraging patient/family member partnerships with the health care team. *Pediatric Nursing*, 38(4), 232–235.

American Academy of Pediatrics (2013). *Types of families*. Retrieved from http://www.healthychildren.org/English/family-life/family-dynamics/types-of-families/Pages/default.aspx

Balick, B., Conway, J., Zipperer, L., & Watson, J. (2011). *Achieving an exceptional patient and family experience of inpatient hospital care.* IHI Innovation Series white paper. Cambridge, MA: Institute for Healthcare Improvement. (Available from http://www.IHI.org).

Benbassat, J., Pilpel, D., & Tidhar, M. (1998). Patients' preferences for participation in clinical decision-making: A review of published surveys. *Behavioral Medicine, 24*(2), 81–88.

Berwick, D. (2009). What "patient-centered" should mean: Confessions of an extremist. *Health Affairs, 28*(4), 555–565.

Burchard, D. J. (2005). Family nursing: Challenges and opportunities: What will the challenges for family nursing be over the next few years? *Journal of Family Nursing, 11*(4), 332–335.

Cannon, S. (2011). Family-centered care in the critical care setting. *Dimensions of Critical Care, 30*(5), 241–245.

Christensen, T. (2007). *Sick girl speaks.* New York: iUniverse.

Corlett, J., & Twycross, A. (2006). Negotiation of parental roles within family-centered care: A review of the research. *Journal of Clinical Nursing, 15*, 1308–1316.

Cook, D. (2001). Patient autonomy versus paternalism. *Critical Care Medicine, 20*(2), N24–N25.

D'Aloja, E., Floris, L., Muller, M., Birocchi, F., Fanos, V., Paribello, F., et al. (2010). Shared decision-making in neonatology: A utopia or an attainable goal? *Journal of Maternal-Fetal Neonatal Medicine, 23* (Suppl 3), 56–8.

Eel, K. (1996). Social networks, social support and coping with serious illness: The family connection. *Social Science Medicine, 42*(2), 173–183.

Espezel, H., & Canam, C. (2003). Parent-nurse interactions: Care of hospitalized children. *Journal of Advanced Nursing, 44*, 34–41.

Feinberg, L. (2012). *Moving toward person-and-family-centered care.* AARP Public Policy Institute. Retrieved from http://www.aarp.org/relationships/caregiving/info-03-2012/moving-toward-person-and-family-centered-care-insight-AARP-ppi-ltc.html

Feinberg, L., Reinhard, S. C., Houser, A., & Choula, R. (2011). *Valuing the invaluable: 2011 update: The growing contributions and costs of family caregiving.* AARP Public Policy Institute. Retrieved from http://assets.aarp.org/rgcenter/ppi/ltc/i51-caregiving.pdf

Frazee, S. (2011). Goal of the day: Initiating goal of the day to improve patient- and family- centered care. *Dimension of Critical Care Nursing, 30*(6), 326–330.

Friedman, M. M. (2002). *Family nursing: Research, theory, and practice* (5th ed.). Stamford, CT: Appleton & Lange.

Hack, T. F., Degner, L. F., Watson, P., & Sinha, L. S. (2005). Do patients benefit from participating in medical decision-making? Longitudinal follow-up of women with breast cancer. *Psycho-Oncology, 15*, 9–19.

Hanson, C. C., & Barach, P. R. (2012). Improving cardiac care quality and safety through partnerships with patients and their families. *Progress in Pediatric Cardiology, 33*, 73–79.

Hawkins, N. A., Pollack, L. A., Leadbetter, S., Steele, W. R., Carrroll, J., Dolan, J. G., et al. (2008). Informational needs of patients and perceived adequacy of information available before and after treatment of cancer. *Journal of Psychosocial Oncology, 26*(2), 1–16.

Henneman, E. A., & Cardin, S. (2002). Family-centered care: A practical approach to making it happen. *Critical Care Nurse, 22*(6), 12–19.

Hunziker, S., McHugh, W., Sarnoff-Lee, B., Cannistraro, S., Marcantonio, E., & Howell, M. D. (2012). Predictors and correlates of dissatisfaction with intensive care. *Critical Care Medicine, 40*(5), 1554–1561.

Institute for Patient- and Family-Centered Care (n.d.a). *Advancing the practice of patient- and family-centered care in hospitals.* Bethesda, MD: Institute for Patient- and Family-Centered Care: Retrieved from http://www.ipfcc.org

Institute for Patient- and Family-Centered Care (n.d.b.). *Advancing the practice of patient- and family-centered care in primary care and other ambulatory care settings.* Bethesda, MD: Institute for Patient- and Family-Centered Care. Retrieved from http://www.ipfcc.org

Institute of Medicine (2001). *Crossing the quality chasm: A new health system for the 21st century.* Washington, DC: National Academies Press.

James, J. (2013, February 14). Health policy brief: patient engagement. *Health Affairs.*

Johnson, B., Abraham, M., Conway, J., Simmons, L., Edgman-Levitan, S., Sodomka, P., et al. (2008). *Partnering with patients and families to design a patient- and family-centered health care system.* Bethesda, MD: Institute for Patient- and Family-Centered Care.

Katz, A. (2012). Editorial. *Oncology Nursing Forum, 39*(4), 331.

Leske, J. S. (1991). Overview of family needs after critical illness: From assessment to intervention. *AACN Clinical Issues Critical Care Nursing, 2*(2), 220–226.

Long, P. (2013). *The patient is in: Listening to low-income Californians.* HealthAffairs Blog. Retrieved from http://healthaffairs.org/blog/2013/02/11/the-patient-is-in-listening-to-low-income-californians

Makoul, G., & Clayman, M. I. (2006). An integrative model of shared decision-making in medical encounters. *Patient Education and Counseling, 60*, 301–312.

Mitchell, M. L., Courney, M., & Coyer, F. (2003). Understanding uncertainty and minimizing families' anxiety at the time of transfer from intensive care. *Nursing and Health Sciences, 5*, 207–217.

National Alliance for Caregiving & AARP. (2009). *Caregiving in the U.S.* Washington, DC: National Alliance for Caregiving. Retrieved from http://www.caregiving.org/data/Caregiving_in_the_US_2009_full_report.pdf

Osborn, T. R., Curtis, J. R., Nielsen, E. L., Beck, A. L., Shannon, S. E., & Engelberg, R. A. (2012). Identifying elements of ICU care that families report as important but unsatisfactory. *Chest, 142*(5), 1185–1192.

Pierce, P. F., & Hicks, F. D. (2001). Patient decision-making behavior. *Nursing Research, 50*(5), 267–274.

Radcliffe, J. J. L., Adeshokan, E. O., Thompson, P. C., & Bakowski, A. J. (2012). Meeting the needs of families and carers on acute psychiatric wards: A nurse-led service. *Journal of Psychiatric and Mental Health Nursing, 19*(8), 751–757.

Salmond, S., & Spears, J. (2002). Psychosocial care of clients and their families. In A. Maher, S. Salmond, & T. Pellino (Eds.), *Orthopaedic nursing* (3rd ed., pp. 26–29). Philadelphia: Saunders.

Sheehan, J., & Sherman, K. A. (2012). Computerised decision aids: A systematic review of their effectiveness in facilitating high-quality decision-making in various health-related contexts. *Patient Education and Counseling, 88*(1), 69–86.

Sobo, E. J. (2004). Pediatric nurses may misjudge parent communication preferences. *Journal of Nursing Care Quality, 19*(3), 253–262.

Stricker, K. H., Kimberger, O., Schmidlin, K., Zwahlen, M., Mohr, U., & Rothen, H. U. (2009). Family satisfaction in the intensive care unit: What makes the difference? *Intensive Care Medicine, 35*(12), 2051–2059.

Taylor, B. (2006). Giving children and parents a voice—The parents' perspective. *Paediatric Nursing, 18*(9), 20–23.

Walton, M. K. (2011). Communicating with family caregivers. *American Journal of Nursing, 111*(12), 47–53.

Warren, N. (2012). Involving patient and family advisors in the patient and family-centered care model. *Medsurg Nursing, 21*(4), 233–239.

World Health Organization (1986). The Ottawa charter for health promotion. Retrieved from http://www.who.int/healthpromotion/conferences/previous/ottawa/en/

Zuo, D. Z., Houtrow, A. J., Arango, P., Kuhlthau, K. A., Simmons, J. M., & Neff, J. M. (2012). Family-centered care: Current applications and future directions in pediatric health care. *Maternal and Child Health Journal, 16*(2), 297–305.

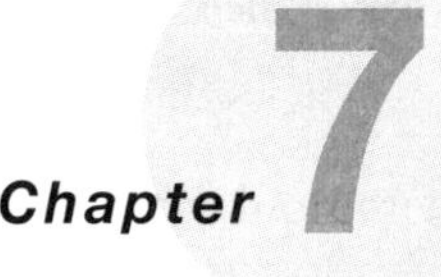

Chapter 7

Media and Decision-Making

Sandy Summers and

Harry Jacobs Summers

Four hostile newspapers are more to be feared than a thousand bayonets.

—Napoleon Bonaparte (1769–1821)

The modern media is pervasive and highly influential. It shapes our culture, our government, and our lives. English statesman Edmund Burke (1739–1797) termed the media the "fourth estate," when he proclaimed its strength greater than all the "three estates in Parliament" (Norris, 2008). Thousands of times every day, the media presents society with a persuasive vision of what society is, what it might be, and what it should be. The media investigates, hosts, and fosters public dialogue, and it regularly influences public decision-making, operating largely outside the domain of government officials in free societies.

The media does more than a government body. The media influences and even creates much of our culture. Its power lies in changing the way people think. U.S. advertisers spend $140 billion per year on advertising (Kantar Media, 2013). Those who spend these vast sums clearly believe that people will take actions based on advertising's persuasive, one-sided flows of information on subjects with which viewers/readers may not have a great deal of prior experience or knowledge. This is also why powerful political ads can move polling numbers and affect election results. In addition, research shows that the news and entertainment media affect what people believe and how they act on a wide range of issues, including health-related issues.

Clearly, the media also has a tremendous impact on how the public sees health care, including nurses and nursing practice. At every moment of every day, the media sends the public powerful messages, not only about important issues like cancer or health insurance, but also about who nurses are, what they know, what they do, and how much their work matters. These messages drive decision-making in all areas and at all levels, including the actions of patients, nurses and their colleagues, hospital managers, top federal officials, and the voters who elect them. The media thus plays a critical role in shaping the current state of nursing care and funding for nursing, and, particularly because the media's overall treatment of nursing is deeply flawed and damaging, it offers important avenues for nurses to improve their situation and the care of their patients.

This chapter starts with a case study that illustrates the media's effect on the population, the image of nurses in the media, and the work that nurses need to do to change that image so that they gain a respected place in healthcare decision-making. The chapter then presents a discussion about how nurses can use the media to increase their visibility, improve their image, and thus become valued decision-makers in health care.

Case Study

In November 2001, as part of the Closing the Health Gap campaign of the U.S. Department of Health and Human Services (HHS), the Office of Minority Health (OMH) launched a new health initiative, the Take a Loved One to the Doctor Day campaign ("Loved One" campaign). The Loved One campaign was cofounded by HHS and ABC Radio's Urban Advantage Network, which had a weekly reach of more than 19 million listeners in 2004 (U.S. Department of Health and Human Services Press Office, 2004). The Loved One campaign's goal was to encourage members of minority populations to take charge of their personal health by educating and empowering them. The campaign is held each year on the third Tuesday of September.

The Loved One campaign soon came to the attention of a small group of graduate students at the Johns Hopkins University School of Nursing. These students had just formed a group called Nursing Vision. The purpose of Nursing Vision was to increase public understanding of nursing and improve media images of nursing, which seemed especially urgent in view of the global nursing shortage. The group was concerned that the U.S. government would be promoting this worthy public health campaign with a name that excluded the work of advanced practice registered nurses (APRNs), who provide a great deal of primary care to the underserved populations that the campaign targets.

When the Loved One issue came to the attention of the Nursing Vision group, members decided to take action. Several members sent letters and made telephone calls to the general number at OMH in early 2002, asking that the Office consider changing the campaign name to one that did not exclude APRNs.

Sandy Summers, Nursing Vision's cofounder, made a call to OMH. She was told that the office would never change the name of the campaign, because the word "doctor" had tested so well in focus groups. After a time, Nursing Vision set the matter aside, concluding that HHS was unlikely to change the name.

Later in 2002, Summers began to work full time on creating a more formal organization to address the widespread misunderstanding of nursing. The group incorporated and became a 501(c)(3) nonprofit organization called the Center for Nursing Advocacy. Summers became the executive director. (In 2008, the Center decided to close and Summers and the other original founding members of Nursing Vision formed a new nonprofit called The Truth About Nursing to continue this work.) In late 2002, the Center launched a Web site on which it analyzed nursing depictions in the media (see TruthAboutNursing.org). Summers also began sending news alerts to supporters and encouraged them to send letters to the media to ask for more accurate depictions of nursing.

Soon, the Center began having some success in convincing corporations to end or modify advertising that used stereotypical images of nurses. A late 2003 *Washington Post* story covered the group's campaign to convince the television show ER to depict nurses more accurately, and that story traveled across the globe (Center for Nursing Advocacy, 2003; Summers & Summers, 2010). With experience and the increase in membership, the Center was becoming more effective.

In October 2004, Summers received a call from the American College of Nurse-Midwives (ACNM). The ACNM remained concerned that the Loved One campaign name reinforced the damaging idea that only physicians provide primary care. Summers decided to renew her efforts to persuade OMH to change the name. The Center was now much larger, and it had a powerful tool at its disposal—a Web page from which a form e-mail letter could be sent. (These were the days before organizations such as Change.org and Care2.org existed that allow anyone to create a letter-writing campaign.) The e-mail form letter tool had been essential to many of the group's other successes.

Summers gathered information. She did research on the Internet, and through calls to OMH collected the names and contact information of high-ranking individuals who would be involved in any decision to rename the campaign. This was a critical advocacy step—finding the real decision-makers—and one that had not been employed in Nursing Vision's initial 2002 efforts.

Summers also collected research comparing the care provided by physicians to the care provided by APRNs (www.truthaboutnursing.org/faq/aprn_md.html). She built a Web page featuring all the studies she found comparing the care of the two groups. The consensus of this research was that care provided by APRNs was as good as or better than that provided by physicians. This research would help to show why the Loved One campaign had no reason to exclude APRNs.

In the meantime, the ACNM drafted a proposed letter to OMH, which it sent to Summers for review in November 2004. In the letter, the ACNM suggested five possible new names for the Loved One campaign, one of which was "Take a Loved One for a Checkup Day." The Center then drafted an analysis of the issue, which explained why the current name of the campaign was so damaging.

With the analysis ready, the Center prepared a letter to be sent to OMH. The Center embraced the ACNM's suggested name change of "Take a Loved One for a Checkup Day." On December 7, 2004, Summers e-mailed the letter to the Assistant Secretary for Minority Health and about seven other people at OMH, as well as the Secretary of HHS, and Tom Joyner, the host of a popular, nationally syndicated urban radio show who had been the honorary co-chair of the Loved One campaign since its inception. Around this same time, ACNM and the American Academy of Nurse Practitioners (AANP) sent their own letters and urged their members to support the Center's campaign to have the name changed; a number of these members visited the Center's Web site and sent letters using the site.

The Center also included a "Take Action" item on the Loved One campaign in its news alert of December 7. The item asked people to write to OMH and the other decision-makers. To make that easier, the item included a link to a proposed e-mail letter that had been adapted from Summers's letter to the decision-makers. Supporters were able to simply sign this form letter, or draft their own letter, and then send the result to the decision-makers from the Center's site. On December 17, Summers issued a press release, but the media failed to pick up the story.

Letters from the Center's Web site began rolling in to HHS from concerned nurses and supporters. The letters appeared to be reaching the e-mail inboxes of at least some of the decision-makers.

A week or two later, in mid-December 2004, Summers called OMH and asked to set up a telephone call with the Assistant Secretary for Minority Health, an executive who was relatively new to the job and had not been with OMH in 2002. By this time, OMH had received about 200 letters from the Center's Web site. After a number of requests, the call was arranged.

On December 21, Summers had a conference call with the Assistant Secretary and another OMH decision-maker. During the call, Summers explained the problem with the "Doctor Day" part of the campaign name and stressed how helpful a change would be. The Assistant Secretary (a physician himself) was receptive, and he agreed to explore the idea of a name change. Summers kept the campaign open, and on January 3, 2005, she sent the Assistant Secretary an e-mail requesting more definitive action on OMH plans to change the "Doctor Day" name so she could end the campaign. Around this time, OMH staff members assured Summers that a letter from the Assistant Secretary would be forthcoming.

On January 12, 2005, American Nurses Association president Barbara Blakeney sent the HHS decision-makers a letter about the name change that was drawn largely from the Center's model.

On January 28, 2005, the Assistant Secretary for Minority Health sent the nursing groups a letter confirming that HHS working groups would seek a new name for the campaign. The Center ended its active campaign about the name. At this point, OMH had received about 370 letters from the Center's Web site.

In July 2005, OMH began issuing materials relating to the upcoming September campaign day. These materials showed that OMH had changed the name to "Take a Loved One for a Checkup Day," as the nursing groups had suggested. The OMH campaign used that name in ensuing years, and almost all of the campaign's media and healthcare partners used the new name as well. Unfortunately, Tom Joyner, the host of the popular syndicated show on ABC Radio's Urban Advantage Network, who continued to serve as honorary co-chair of the campaign, refused to use the new name. His office dismissed the nurses' concerns, telling Summers in a phone call that the change could have "harmful effects" and that the original name had "capital." In recent years, OMH has not played a major role in the campaign. And presumably because of Joyner's ongoing insistence on calling it "Doctor Day," that name has again become more common, although some groups

Figure 7-1

A "Loved One" campaign ad, with name changed.

GOOD
HEALTH
NEEDS
HELP
Start with a checkup
Take a Loved One for
a Checkup Day

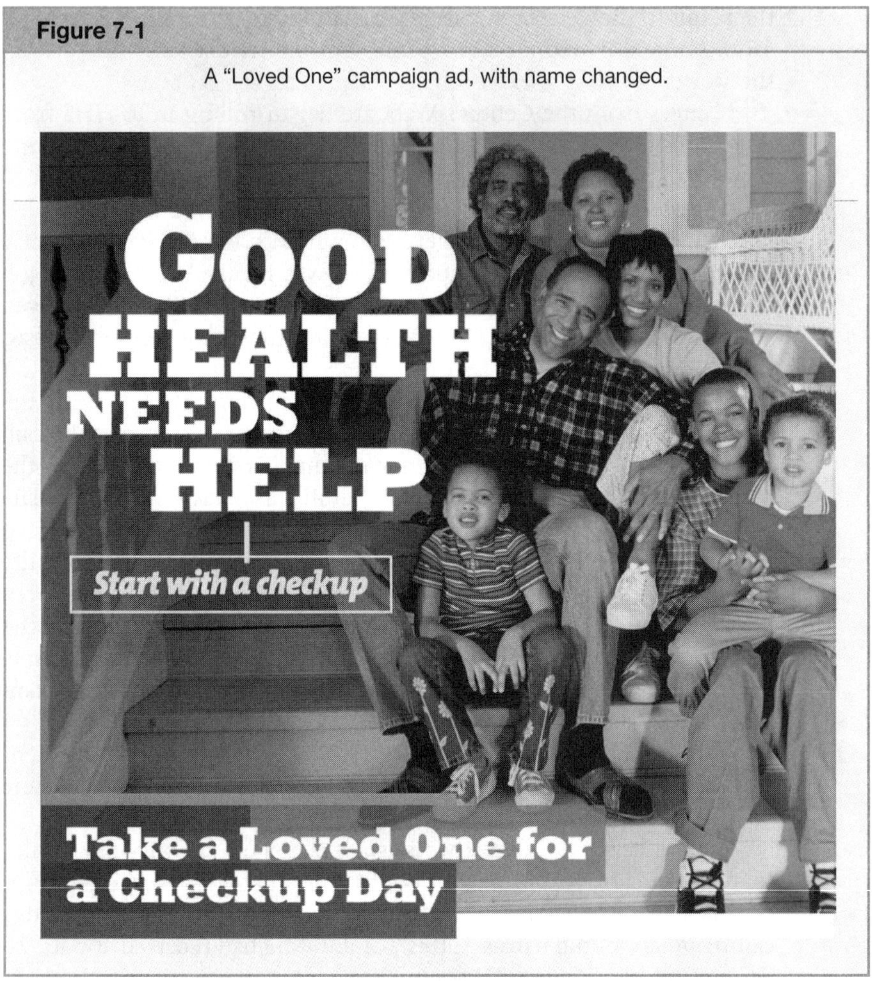

Source: U.S. Department of Health and Human Services.

still use "Checkup Day." Working for universal buy-in of the "Checkup Day" name continues to be an important goal for The Truth About Nursing. Join the campaign at www.TruthAboutNursing.org/joyner. (See **Figure 7-1**.)

This case study is an example of how one small group decided to take action and place constructive pressure on a second very powerful group. This pressure, applied via the use of media strategies, caused a shift in the second group's perceptions, resulting in a decision to change the name of a prominent national media campaign. The tactics used may be applied in any venue where the message of the media would help effect positive change. The change in the title of this media campaign gave the public greater awareness of and thus access to healthcare providers other than the doctor, and it potentially improved understanding of the value of nurses and their ability to be included as decision makers in health care.

The Pervasive Influence of the Media

The average American spends 11.8 hours per day, or 70 percent of each person's awake time, consuming information (Bohn & Short, 2012; eMarketer, 2012). Research shows that this media—including advertising and entertainment programming—has a significant impact on what consumers think and do. Nurses therefore have an enormous opportunity to bring messages about nursing and health care generally to patients and society at large by tapping into the insatiable desire for media entertainment and information. Unfortunately, although there have been accurate and helpful depictions of nursing, too much of the media's depiction of the profession has been damaging. This poor depiction affects the public's ideas about the value of nursing, and about nurses' role and influence in healthcare decision-making.

Effects of Media on Health Care and Nursing

In recent years, a consensus has emerged in the field of public health, based on considerable research, that what people see in the media has a significant effect on their health-related views and behavior. A wide range of public agencies, private groups, and scholars now devote substantial resources to analyzing and managing health messages in the media. This is part of the public health field called *health communication*.

Health communication is a hybrid, with roots in communications, health care, and other fields (Glik, 2003). Glik (2003) states that health communications contain both planned and unplanned messages that can be positive, neutral, or negative. These unplanned messages are significant in that people are influenced by media content whether or not the creators specifically intended that they take away the message received. In recent years, the field of health communication has gained prominence (Rimal & Lapinsky, 2009), and health communication scholars have recognized the growing impact of new media on the public's understanding of key health issues (Parker & Thorson, 2009).

What the media tells people about health care works much like advertising. As one public health scholar noted, "from a social marketing perspective, messages in the media that promote specific desirable behaviors have the potential to persuade consumers to change their behavior if messages are viewed as compatible with consumers' own self-interest, competing messages are minimal, and resistance to change is low to moderate" (Glik, 2003, p. 1).

News media coverage also affects the public's perception and beliefs about health care (Turow & Gans, 2002). Because treatment of health topics in the news media has a significant effect on public views and actions, advocates have worked hard to affect the frequency and accuracy of the media's coverage of health topics in which they have an interest (Glik, 2003).

Media influence is hardly confined to hard-news outlets. On the contrary, what people see in entertainment media also has a significant effect on their health-related views and behavior, as public health leaders recognize. For example, each summer from 2003 to 2007, the Robert Wood Johnson Foundation expressed its concern about how physicians were portrayed on television by distributing copies of scholar Joseph Turow's DVD essay *Prime Time Doctors: Why Should You Care?* to about 20,000 U.S. medical students (Herman, 2013).

Research has confirmed the influence of entertainment television. In 2000, the U.S. Centers for Disease Control and Prevention surveyed prime-time TV viewers and found that most (52 percent) reported getting information that they trust to be accurate from prime-time TV shows (Henry J. Kaiser Family Foundation, 2004). More than a quarter of this survey's respondents said such shows were among their top three sources for health information (Henry J. Kaiser, 2004). Nine out of 10 regular viewers said they learned something about diseases or disease prevention from television, with almost half citing prime-time or daytime entertainment shows (Henry J. Kaiser, 2004). Moreover, almost half of regular viewers who heard something about a health issue on a prime-time show said they took one or more actions, including telling someone about the storyline (42 percent), telling someone to do something (such as using a condom or getting more exercise) or doing it themselves (16 percent), or visiting a clinic (9 percent) (Henry J. Kaiser, 2004). A study published in the journal *Plastic and Reconstructive Surgery* found that reality shows played an important role in patients' knowledge of and decisions about plastic surgery (Crockett, Pruzinsky, & Persing, 2007).

Some research has focused on the effects of specific shows, including the popular, long-running dramas *ER* (NBC) and *Grey's Anatomy* (ABC). *ER* aired new episodes from 1994 to 2009 and has been shown in many nations around the world; it continues to air in syndication. During the U.S. television seasons running during 1997–2000, the Henry J. Kaiser Family Foundation surveyed 3,500 regular *ER* viewers (Brodie et al., 2001; Henry J. Kaiser, 2002, 2003). In the Kaiser surveys, more than half (53 percent) of regular *ER* viewers said they learned about important health issues while watching the show. Almost a third said information from the show helped them make choices about their own family's health care; this was especially true of viewers with less formal education (44 percent with no college versus 25 percent with some college). As a result of watching *ER*, almost a quarter of viewers said they sought further information about a health issue, and 14 percent actually contacted a healthcare provider because of something they saw in an *ER* episode. In addition, a 2009 University of Alberta study published in *Resuscitation* found that many residents and medical students had learned incorrect intubation techniques by watching *ER* and other shows (Brindley & Needham, 2009).

Recent research has shown that *Grey's Anatomy*, which first aired in 2005, likewise affects how the public sees health care. In 2008, the Kaiser Family Foundation released a study showing that an embedded *Grey's* plotline about maternal HIV transmission had significantly increased audience understanding of the issue. The show's director of medical research helped to publicize the study and reportedly stated that the show took its influence "very seriously" (Rideout, 2008).

Other studies have suggested a link between entertainment media and public attitudes toward nursing in particular. In a 2000 JWT Communications focus group study of youngsters in grades 2–10, respondents said they received their main impression of nursing from *ER* (JWT Communications, 2000). Consistent with the show's physician-centric approach, the young people also wrongly believed that nursing was a girl's job, that it was a technical job "like shop," and that it was an inappropriate career for private school students, of whom more was expected (JWT Communications, 2000).

A 2008 University of Dundee (Scotland) study found that media imagery discouraged academically advanced primary school students from nursing careers by presenting nurses as, in the words of one student, "brainless, sex-mad bimbos" looking to "romance" physicians. Consistent with the earlier JWT research, the Dundee study found that the students' main source of images about nursing was television. Based on all imagery, the students concluded that becoming a nurse would not be "using their examination grades to maximum benefit" (Neilson & Lauder, 2008).

Finally, in 2012, a study at University College Dublin (Ireland) found that the most popular videos posted on the YouTube Web site stereotype nurses as stupid and/or sex objects. The researchers found that of the 10 most popular nurse-related YouTube videos, four portrayed nurses as sex objects, two showed nurses as stupid or incompetent, and only four—all posted by nurses themselves—showed nursing as a skilled and caring profession. All six of the stereotypical depictions were from television products or ads (Kelly, Fealy, & Watson, 2012).

Nursing's Role in Shaping Health Messages

Nurses can help to shape health messages for public consumption. However, the profession's public image may actually impede nurses' efforts to play this role.

Although nurses commonly top polls measuring which professions are the most ethical and honest, any serious evaluation of the profession's public image reveals that most people do not understand what nurses actually do or why nursing work matters (The Truth About Nursing, 2012a). On the contrary, nursing's public image has long been based primarily on stereotypes, including the physician's handmaiden, the angel, and the naughty nurse (Summers & Summers, 2010; Kalisch & Kalisch, n.d.; Kalisch & Kalisch, 1986, n.d.). Although nurses have tended to enjoy public affection, they have not received the real respect that might lead to a better allocation of clinical, educational, and research resources for the profession or allow nurses a real seat at the table of policy making and clinical decision-making. Nurses' image as workers without significant knowledge also has negatively affected the public's perception of the validity of information that nurses offer them for health decision-making, both on an individual basis and in wider public forums. To take just one example, consider the primitive depictions of family presence on television dramas, which regularly feature physicians ordering family members far away from patient bedsides during emergency procedures as a matter of course, as if no one had ever questioned this practice. If nurses had meaningful input, it seems likely that such influential shows would be giving the public a better sense of evolving health practices in this regard (The Truth About Nursing, 2009; Center for Nursing Advocacy, 2006a).

Because research shows that the media has such a strong influence on public understanding of nursing and health care in general, it is vital to nursing and public health that nurses improve their media image. Indeed, if the mass media is critical to modern health strategies overall, then it must also be a key means of addressing one of the most important worldwide health problems: the nursing shortage. Although the number of open nursing *positions* in the United States has declined as a result of the Great Recession, the shortage of global nursing *care* as a result of understaffing remains a critical issue (Donnelly, 2012; Sapatkin, 2012).

Media Portrayal of Nurses: The Stereotypes

The media frequently portrays nursing work because nursing involves life, death, conflict, and drama—the stuff of compelling and important media. Unfortunately, the media commonly portrays nurses stereotypically, often crediting physicians for nursing work, and this is especially true of the most influential form of media—television. Factors contributing to this may include entrenched social biases (including gender bias) and assumptions about nursing, including:

- The view that smart, ambitious women with an interest in health care necessarily become physicians
- What one scholar has called *nursism*, a more general social bias against the caring role that contributes negatively to the way nursing is perceived (Lewenson, 1993)
- The media's common reliance on well-understood (but often incorrect) conventions
- A lack of significant support for nursing from the physicians who continue to exercise great influence over the media and who enjoy unparalleled esteem, including the widespread assumption that they provide all important health care
- Nursing's own failure to adequately represent itself to the media and the public at large

There have been notable exceptions, particularly in the print media, documentaries, and a few fictional products (The Truth About Nursing, 2012b). However, the overall impression of nursing the public gets from the media is distorted and inadequate to the needs of nurses and their patients.

The most common nursing stereotypes are:

- *The physician handmaiden:* Nurses have long been portrayed as fungible females who have no great level of training, no unique scope of practice, and no significant role in substantive health care. Instead, they are seen to exist to help the physicians who do provide important health care; it is assumed that physicians supervise and manage nurses and know everything nurses do. This is perhaps the most damaging stereotype, because it remains so common and so persuasive to a public that knows little of what nurses really do. Indeed, the handmaiden remains the central nursing image in popular Hollywood television shows, where the few nurses who appear seem to exist to get physicians or get things for physicians. Handmaiden images range from the less-obviously damaging portrayals of nurses as skilled physician subordinates, as seen on shows like *ER*, to the explicit attacks on the profession in products like *Grey's Anatomy* or *House* (Fox), where nurses tend to be clueless, often disagreeable servants who represent everything ambitious modern women have left behind (Summers & Summers, 2010). The nurse-focused shows introduced in 2009, notably the powerful *Nurse Jackie* (Showtime) but also the more short-lived *Mercy* (NBC) and *HawthoRNe* (TNT), often portrayed nurses as skilled professionals who saved lives and even, at times, worked autonomously. In many instances, though, even these shows presented nurse characters as reporting to physicians. Ironically, the recent U.K. drama *Call the Midwife* (PBS), although set in the 1950s, has generally done a better job of portraying nurses working autonomously (The Truth About Nursing, 2010, 2011a, 2012c, 2012d).

- *The naughty nurse:* The naughty nurse image commonly takes the form of a female model or actress dressed in a supposed "nursing uniform" that amounts to lingerie. Such images remain a staple of media communications of the advertising, apparel, hospitality, and entertainment industries, particularly in products directed at younger males. Some entertainment programming continues to suggest that nurses tend to be sexually available to physicians or patients. Examples include the depiction of "skanky syph[ilis] nurse" Olivia on *Grey's Anatomy*, and the appearance of the lead character as a naughty nurse on a 2011 episode of the sitcom *Whitney* (NBC). Even physician Mehmet Oz, in a 2010 segment on his globally popular syndicated television show, danced with provocatively attired "nurses" to promote dancing as a weight loss tactic. (After The Truth About Nursing launched a campaign, he publicly apologized.) The Truth About Nursing (in efforts similar to those discussed in the earlier case study) has convinced many media creators to reconsider such images, though the images continue to appear in prominent media worldwide. As The Truth has explained, even though these images are often "jokes" or "fantasies," the stereotypes they promote discourage practicing and potential nurses, foster sexual violence in the workplace, and contribute to a general atmosphere of disrespect that makes it difficult for nurses to get the respect and resources they need (Summers & Summers, 2010).
- *The angel:* On the surface, the image of nurses as angels seems to be the best of the stereotypes, and some nurses themselves endorse it. Indeed, the angel image is fueled by some media products that are designed to appeal to nurses, such as uniforms. However, the image of nurses as devoted hand-holders and scut-work saints undervalues nurses' knowledge and advanced skills. It may also allow decision makers to discount poor working conditions that nurses endure or to treat the conditions as evidence of nurses' virtue, rather than problems that must be addressed (Summers & Summers, 2010). We view most of the Johnson & Johnson Campaign for Nursing's Future television commercials as employing this stereotype. A trusted, baby-soft image is obviously helpful to a major pharmaceutical corporation, which benefits by aligning itself with a profession

that the public sees as the most ethical and honest, but nursing itself is not well-served by the view that nurses are relatively unskilled spiritual beings with no earthly needs (The Truth About Nursing, 2011b).

- *The battle-ax:* The battle-ax image essentially presents the nurse as an unattractive, bitter, and malevolent force, often the representation of an unfeeling bureaucracy or institutional oppression. This image continues to appear from time to time in advertising and entertainment programming. The image may stem in part from a need to compensate for a feeling that female nurses may have significant power over vulnerable men in clinical settings, and from a belief that any assertive nurse who fails to conform to the more submissive nursing stereotypes must be a she-demon. Nurse Ratched from the book and film *One Flew Over the Cuckoo's Nest* is perhaps the best-known example of the battle-ax, a portrayal that may be the most influential modern image of a nurse who seems to delight in torturing patients. A newer variant is what The Truth About Nursing calls the "naughty-ax," a character who combines sexual aggressiveness with malevolence. The Margaret "Hot Lips" Houlihan character in the film and television series M*A*S*H at times hinted at this toxic mix, but recent examples have been more extreme, particularly in horror films such as *Silent Hill: Revelation 3D* (2012), which was based on a popular video game series (Summers & Summers, 2010).
- *The physician gold digger:* This image has long existed in tandem with the strand of the naughty nurse image that presents the nurse as being sexually available to physicians. For example, in 2004, television psychologist Dr. Phil McGraw suggested on the air that the healthcare system is full of "cute little nurses" who are out to "seduce and marry" physicians "because that's their ticket out of having to work as a nurse." Dr. Phil later made on-air statements expressing support for nursing after Sandy Summers contacted the show and the show received more than 1,400 letters sent through the Center for Nursing Advocacy's Web site (Center for Nursing Advocacy, 2004a).
- *The female caregiver:* Even a casual look at the preceding images shows that the most common nursing stereotypes are closely linked to the prevailing assumption that nurses are female caregivers. In the JWT Communications (2000) research of 1,800 U.S. schoolchildren in grades 2–10, researchers found that when the focus groups' topic changed to nursing, the boys stopped paying attention, as if the conversation no longer pertained to them. And the University College Dublin researchers who did the 2012 YouTube study noted that the most popular videos they found presented nurses as female (Kelly et al., 2012).

- It has been persuasively argued that caregiving has long been admired, but rarely considered intellectually challenging or truly essential outside of the family structure (Nelson & Gordon, 2006). Although there has been recent media coverage about men in nursing and a few minor nurse characters in recent Hollywood shows have been male, major depictions of nurses remain overwhelmingly female. Of course, nursing does remain less than 10 percent male (U.S. Department of Health and Human Services, 2010). However, as long as nursing is portrayed as a profession for "caring" females, it will be considered work that is too effeminate and insubstantial for men—and too lowly for anyone interested in an autonomous, challenging career (Summers & Summers, 2010).
- *Any helpful person or thing is a nurse:* The media has tended to suggest that nursing is something any caring person can do—that any caregiver is a "nurse." Consider the recent growth in "baby nurses," who are actually nannies for newborns who may have no healthcare training at all. Still, these workers commonly refer to themselves—and are referred to in the major media—by the shorthand "nurse." After one "baby nurse" allegedly injured a newborn in New York in 2005, the state legislature passed a law to prevent nonnurses from calling themselves "nurses" (Center for Nursing Advocacy, 2005a). In 2006, the CVS pharmaceutical chain produced a television commercial in which a pharmacist suggested that by helping a patient's spouse learn about her complex medication regimen in half a day, he had turned the spouse into a nurse. After a few calls from us, CVS removed this statement from its commercial (Center for Nursing Advocacy, 2006b). Another common version of this image appears when makers of electronic healthcare tools that perform relatively simple tasks market their products with names like "electronic nurse" or otherwise suggest that the product will be acting as a nurse, as has been the case with some surgical robots. The Center for Nursing Advocacy has convinced some of these creators to stop naming their products after skilled nurses (Center for Nursing Advocacy, 2006c); however, the media is often eager to call the machines "nurses." For example, in 2011, an Associated Press item reported that Purdue University researchers were developing a "robotic scrub nurse" that could recognize five hand gestures (The Truth About Nursing, 2011c).
- *The wallpaper nurse:* Nurse characters populate the background of popular television shows like *Grey's Anatomy*, doing busy work as a kind of garnish to the glamorous, important work of the heroic physicians on which the camera focuses. These "wallpaper nurses" may morph out of the background to push gurneys,

deliver messages, or hand things to physicians. They often are presented as mute automatons who would seem not to need significant education or resources; certainly few viewers would want to see themselves in such a role. Ironically, the actors playing these roles are often real nurses (Summers & Summers, 2010).

- *The physician nurse:* Physician characters on fictional television shows are often presented performing the work that real-life nurses do. There were about 55 major physician characters but only about 7 nurses on the health-related U.S. primetime shows airing in the 2012–2013 season. And five of those nurse characters were on *Nurse Jackie*. Because the majority of real hospital work is done by nurses, including tasks involving patient interactions and many of the key tasks in critical procedures, the media's physician characters must perform the work of nurses just to make the shows' drama work. This effectively gives physicians credit for the exciting work that nurses really do. At the same time, the news media commonly consults only physicians for advice in areas where nurses generally have greater expertise, such as breastfeeding, pain management, and patient education (Summers & Summers, 2010).
- *The cut-rate physician substitute:* A large body of research shows that the care of Advanced Practice Registered Nurses (APRNs) is at least as good as that provided by physicians (The Truth About Nursing, 2011d), yet media entities often present items that ignore the very existence of APRNs, even in areas where APRNs play a central role, such as primary care for underserved populations. As noted in the case study at the beginning of the chapter, in 2005 nurses persuaded the U.S. Department of Health and Human Services to change the name of its annual minority health campaign from "Take a Loved One to the Doctor Day" to "Take a Loved One for a Checkup Day" (Center for Nursing Advocacy, 2005b). The news media may also accept criticism of APRN care by competitors in organized medicine with little or no question, as has often occurred in connection with the growth of APRN-staffed retail-based clinics. Such press pieces often do not even consult APRNs or the organizations that represent them (Summers & Summers, 2010).

The prevalence of these stereotypes has a significant negative impact on healthcare decision-making and nursing. When nurses are seen mainly as low-skilled physician subordinates, their healthcare expertise has less impact on colleagues, patients, the media, and the public. Nurses also struggle to get the resources they need to provide high-quality direct care, to conduct vital research, and to educate a new generation of nurses.

The Challenge of Getting "Real Nursing" into the Media

The question remains: How do we get real nursing into the media, so we can change the population's perception of nursing? This is essential if the voice of nursing in the shaping of health care is to be heard, especially as the nation moves to implement the Affordable Care Act of 2010 and the recommendations to strengthen nursing practice in the Institute of Medicine's (2010) landmark report *The Future of Nursing*. At the very least, it is important that patients value nurses' advice and apply it in day-to-day health decision-making. To improve public understanding of nursing and improve health care itself, nurses must become more involved in shaping the media that the public consumes—yet getting nursing into the media is a monumental challenge. Nurses have been reluctant to step forward and reach out to the media. At the same time, the media has failed to seek out nurses for their expert comment, instead consulting physicians on subjects for which nurses are generally more expert. This is presumably a result of the cumulative effect of the stereotypical nursing image just discussed, but it may stem in particular from the belief that nursing is merely a minor subset of medicine, rather than a distinct, autonomous profession (The Truth About Nursing, 2013). When nurses have so little independent credibility in the media, it is hard for them to be seen as reliable, knowledgeable health resources by their patients and the wider public (Summers & Summers, 2010).

The Process of Communicating

In mass communication, there is typically a sender, a message, a recipient, and feedback (Reynolds, 1997). The message is crafted to reach certain types of recipients; often, it is aimed at a specific demographic. The message is sent in a specific medium, with the sender making an effort to cut through background noise and clutter. Recipients decode the message in their own way based on the message, the clutter, and the level of credibility of the sender, which affects whether recipients take action on the message in accord with the sender's goals (Freed, 2006).

Under this framework, nurses who wish to communicate must assess their credibility as health educators. Of course, it is often said that Gallup polls show nurses have a high level of public "trust," although the polls actually measure "ethics and honesty" (Gallup, 2012). But trust in a person's ethics and honesty is not the same as respect for that person's autonomy and professional skill. Based on the rampant negative media depictions and relatively low funding for the nursing profession as a whole, it seems that the public trusts nurses to hold their wallets while they are in surgery, but does not trust nurses to play a significant role in keeping patients alive while they are actually in surgery or to educate them about how to recover. True respect for the profession would entail meaningful public inquiry into the nature of nursing work and the people who do it. It would mean serious governmental funding to address the global nursing shortage—one of the greatest ongoing public health crises in today's world. If the entire world had a ratio of 1 nurse for every 100 citizens, as some developed nations do, we would need 70 million nurses, *five times the number we have now*. True respect would mean including nurses on every board and committee related to health. It would mean that at least half of every hospital board was composed of nurses; after all, hospitals are nursing institutions—they should be run primarily by nurses. However, because nursing is undervalued, these things are not happening.

The bedrock components of nursing practice are direct patient care, patient education, and patient advocacy. Nursing education, nursing research, and nursing advocacy underpin each of the three components. When nurses advocate for a stronger profession, they are improving their direct care and their ability to educate and advocate for patients. If nurses wish to increase the number of people who take positive action based on their health messages, they must increase their credibility as health educators—and that begins with improving their media image.

If nurses continue to avoid participating in the media, they will miss vital opportunities to reach patients and society with key health information, including information to help the public better understand nursing itself. Patients will lack the information they need to make good health decisions. In recent years, some nurses have worked effectively to communicate about their work, through media such as books, radio shows, op-ed pieces, and public advocacy campaigns (The Truth About Nursing, 2012c). However, the profession must be far more vocal and assertive if it is to make the sea of change in public understanding that the current situation requires.

Nurses Must Improve Nursing's Image in Order to Improve Health Care

Some might ask why nurses have to improve the nursing image in order to get key health messages to patients and the public. The reason is that when nursing is so undervalued in the public consciousness—when people think that only physicians have substantive knowledge about health issues—then patients do not hear or act upon nurses' health messages.

Consider the last time you were at a family gathering, neighborhood cookout, or party. It is common for nurses to meet new people or old friends and have the conversation turn to careers or personal health issues. In such situations, nurses have a great opportunity to educate people, one by one, about the work of nursing and health issues—both of which would establish nurses as health experts. Family, friends, or acquaintances might tell a nurse of their health concerns, and particularly given nursing's strong focus on preventative health and health management, the nurse might be eager to educate as well as possible given the social setting. However, many nurses report that social bias or nursism can work against them in these settings. Nurses often have the sense that their messages are not heard, believed, or adopted, even though they are based on evidence and years of advanced training, particularly if the nursing advice appears to be inconsistent with that of a physician.

It would hardly take a logical leap to surmise that the basic reason for this lack of perceived credibility is the huge gulf in the levels of genuine social respect for medicine and nursing. Because nurses are constantly seen as people who do not know anything meaningful or substantive, their expert advice is often ignored or discounted—and needless to say, this problem exists in clinical settings as well; nurses often have the sense that what they tell patients and non-nurse colleagues is discounted in critical decision-making. However, neither patients nor colleagues can afford to undervalue nurses' teaching. It is vital to public health that these recipients hear and heed nurses' messages, many of which the recipients are unlikely to hear anywhere else—and many of which could make the difference between life and death.

If nurses want to reach out to the media and start affecting it, they need to know the nuts and bolts of how the media works. As psychologist Kurt Lewin (1890–1947) said: "If you want to truly understand something, try to change it" (Kwantlen Polytechnic University, n.d.). What follows are suggestions to do just this, using the media as a way to educate the populations that nurses serve in their own everyday decision-making.

Every nurse should read and consider the advice in *From Silence to Voice* by Bernice Buresh and Suzanne Gordon (2006). The authors are experienced journalists who explain how the media works and how nurses can better participate in media coverage. This important book shows that nurses have not given the public an adequate account of their work, but it offers strategies to help nurses tell the world what they do, in order to get the resources and respect needed to resolve the nursing crisis and help patients achieve better health.

Interested nurses should also read the excellent sixth edition (2011) of *Policy and Politics in Nursing and Health Care*, edited by Diana Mason, Judith Leavitt, and Mary Chaffee. Especially helpful is Chapter 10, "Role of Media in Influencing Policy: Getting the Message Across," which features information on getting free media coverage that establishes nurses as health experts.

Nurses who believe they may have the opportunity to speak to the media should consider getting media training. Nurses' employers can encourage such training, and perhaps pay for the costs, in order to help nurses increase understanding of their work and promote the institution by extension. In fact, institutions might consider maintaining a core group of nurses who are skilled at interacting with the media. The Truth About Nursing's media-training resources page, www.truthaboutnursing.org/action/media_training.html, has links to discussions of media myths, media training seminars and workshops, and online resources. Nurses can also get tips on writing powerful letters in The Truth About Nursing's guide at www.truthaboutnursing.org/action/get_help_writing.html.

The following are some specific strategies nurses might use to persuade society that they and their messages are worthy of attention.

Reach Out to the Media

To get media coverage, nurses must actively seek it. As Buresh and Gordon (2006) show, nurses have traditionally shied away from the media in accord with the prevailing "virtue script," which entails a code of self-effacement. Naturally, physicians and others have been happy to supply the media with input that nurses have declined to provide. This system has not served the profession of nursing well, so nurses must work to make sure they are seen and heard.

Appoint a Public Relations Professional to Promote Nursing

One way to get the word out about the work that nurses do at an institution is to appoint a public relations (PR) person who is dedicated solely to that task. Many hospitals have one or more PR professionals who promote physicians and the hospital in general, but there is rarely a focus on nursing. However, Massachusetts General Hospital (MGH) has a PR person dedicated to promoting only nursing at the hospital. Other hospitals should be encouraged to follow this example. In October 2005, the *Boston Globe* published an excellent four-part, front-page series on the training of a new ICU nurse. In order to get the story, the *Globe* reporter and photographer spent 9 months following a veteran nurse and her apprentice at MGH. That article was the result of significant effort by MGH's PR director for nursing Georgia Peirce, who spent months convincing the *Globe* to follow nurses and report on their work (Center for Nursing Advocacy, 2005c).

Provide News Resources for the Media

Individual nurses should offer to serve as expert resources for the media. In doing so, nurses should take care to be responsive, reliable, and credible. Specific measures nurses might consider to do this more effectively include:

- Collecting and promoting story ideas to help the media develop stories on nursing, and incorporate a nursing perspective in general healthcare stories
- Building a database of information on local nursing issues to use as a resource for responding to media inquiries
- Creating a roster of nurses who are expert in different fields to have on hand when the media does ask for expert input
- Developing online video news programs or Web sites that depict real images of nursing
- Determining who a media entity's gatekeeper or decision maker is, and arranging to speak to that person
- Issuing press releases that create a framework for a story about nursing and health

One impressive example of this kind of media outreach is the work of the *American Journal of Nursing* (*AJN*) that began under the leadership of former editor-in-chief Diana J. Mason. *AJN* has done a great job of communicating with the general media about nursing research and other material appearing in the journal. *AJN* has created press releases about significant material it runs and has regularly contacted the media to pitch stories of interest. A compelling narrative story from *AJN* was republished in the November 2004 *Reader's Digest*, with readership of more than 100 million (Reader's Digest Association, 2011). The story told how one nurse spurred a declining leukemia patient's recovery after a bone marrow transplant by subtly getting him to engage with her over a cup of tea (Center for Nursing Advocacy, 2004b). The type of media outreach *AJN* has done is the method used by physician journals, which is one reason their research receives such widespread press coverage.

Create Media with Accurate Depictions of Nurses

Nurses must develop media that gives the public an accurate vision of the profession, including both its achievements and its problems. Many types of media can reach out to patients and educate them about health topics or nursing. For example, advertising can be very effective, especially when there is a good match among the medium, the message, and the resources of the advertiser. Television is a powerful way to communicate basic ideas, but it can be expensive unless a broadcaster donates the airtime. It appears to be easier to get donated radio airtime as compared to television. In 2013, the Ad Council reported donations of radio, television, and cable airtime, together with space in newspapers and other media, with a total value of $1.8 billion. Major newspapers and other publications can reach a significant audience with more complex messages, but they can be expensive. Radio and the Internet may be more affordable ways to reach certain audiences.

Society needs to know that nurses are experts in clinical practice and in health education. Potential ways to advance those goals include health education videos, articles, books (fiction and nonfiction), short stories, guides, television shows, movies (features, shorts, documentaries, animated), novels, plays, poems, Web sites, radio programs, paintings, comics, cartoons, children's interactive CDs, children's books, children's videos, coloring books, Halloween costumes, dolls, action figures, toys, and board games. Although such media might help to interest career seekers, the profession also needs nurses to create media that presents the challenges and problems that nursing confronts today. See more on creating nursing media at www.truthaboutnursing.org/create/.

An example of a paid advertising campaign with major television and Internet components is Johnson & Johnson's prominent Campaign for Nursing's Future, whose stated goal has been to increase interest in nursing careers. Some elements of this campaign, particularly the campaign's Web site and a short video about nurse scientists, contain helpful and persuasive information. As discussed earlier, the campaign's more influential television advertising spots tend to reinforce angel and handmaiden imagery, but Johnson & Johnson has cited research suggesting that its campaign has significantly raised the profile of nursing in certain segments of the community and helped to increase interest in nursing careers (Stringer, 2012).

Of course, shaping the course of existing media activity (paid and unpaid) remains critical because of the media's vast influence, and the fact that it constantly portrays health care, including nurses and nursing. The work of nursing so often is the subject of media attention because it is dramatic and exciting, filled with both intense emotion and cutting-edge technology, life and death, hope and despair. Influencing this media is often the most effective and affordable way to affect the nursing image and to deliver key health messages. Moreover, one of the best ways to advance any cause is earned media—press that those with a given interest generate by doing newsworthy things and encouraging the press to cover them. Of course, media created by those who are not seen to share a specific policy agenda (such as advancing nursing or some health message) can have more credibility with the public. Nurses can make claims about their work, but what the public sees about nursing in major newspapers (or Hollywood dramas) may be taken as a more objective account of the profession.

Although shaping existing media activity does not require direct payments, it can require a tremendous expenditure of time, effort, and skill, as evidenced by the case study presented at the beginning of the chapter. It can take years and more to make a change. The media rarely approaches nurses and asks them how it should portray them or health care generally. Therefore, nurses must work for better treatment of the health issues that matter to them.

Present a Professional Image of Nursing

Before nurses can expect to improve nursing's image, they must examine the image that each of them presents to the world. Some nurses may think professionalism means conforming to a traditional ideal of appearance, such as the white-starched apron and cap. Others may adopt a strict approach toward colleagues, patients, and families, imposing needless restrictions to maintain order, yet many professionals would not define their professions in these terms, but in terms of an unflagging commitment to the best interests of those they serve.

Part of any profession's image relates to the appearance of its members, and this may be particularly true for groups that do not enjoy automatic respect. If nurses want respect, they should strive to look like college-educated science professionals, as physicians and others in the clinical setting do. Some nurses wear patterned scrubs, and of course, the media often portrays nurses as doing so. One 2006 episode of ER presented a resident physician who was mortified that, because her usual clothes had become messy at the hospital, she had to change into patterned scrubs that made her look like a nurse. Unsurprisingly, she was mocked by another physician. Many feel that patterned scrubs say, "Disrespect me!" to the public, just as the similar-looking 1960s housedresses said about homemakers.

Another important element of nurses' professional appearance is recognition in clinical settings that a nurse actually is a nurse. This is especially important because of the recent proliferation of other hospital workers, particularly unlicensed assistive personnel who may, unfortunately, be assigned nursing tasks. Nurses need to take ownership of their own image, and it is not in the profession's interest for nurses to be confused with others in the clinical setting. Nurses should consider wearing the "RN" patch created in 2003 by Mark Dion and J. Morgan Puett, in collaboration with the Fabric Workshop and Museum in Philadelphia. The Truth About Nursing makes available various versions of the RN patch for nurses with different educational credentials to help teach patients (and remind fellow health professionals) that it takes rigorous education to become a nurse. See more on uniforms and the RN patches at www.truthaboutnursing.org/patches.

Nurses and others should also consider what messages their choice of language may send. When we suggest "nurse-friendly" language, we of course do not mean language that is nice to nurses, but language that reflects recognition that nurses are highly skilled health professionals who save lives and improve outcomes. (Similarly, "user-friendly" does not mean language that is nice to users in some generic sense, but language that promotes understanding.) The nurse-friendly language section on The Truth About Nursing's Web site encourages the use of language that sends an accurate message about nurses and their role in health care. Some questions tackled are: Are nurses who don't work at the bedside "real nurses"? Should we refer to physician or nurse practitioner care plans as "orders" (or prescriptions)? See more on nurse-friendly language at www.truthaboutnursing.org/faq/nf/.

Nursing's Influence on the Healthcare Decisions of Others

If nurses succeed in reducing the impact of the current stereotypes of their profession, nurses' voices will increasingly be recognized for what they are, and not seen as the natterings of some degraded fictional vision of nursing. Nurses then will be seen as valuable and reliable sources of information who can guide others in making important health decisions.

However, nurses must keep in mind that engaging with health-related media entails both opportunities and responsibilities. If the lay media is currently covering a health story or piece of research, people are very likely to start asking health professionals about it.

Three in five adults have used the Internet to research health issues (Pew Internet & American Life Project, 2010). Some Internet-educated patients ask nurses probing questions about diseases or other health topics. Nurses must make efforts to stay connected to the information that the individuals they serve are accessing, so that nurses are conversant with new developments and able to respond to questions and concerns. Of course, it can be dangerous to rely on a lay media reporter's interpretation of a healthcare study, so nurses should go straight to the original research when getting health information to make sure they understand and can explain it to patients better. Lay media articles almost always include the name of the underlying resource—usually a published article in a healthcare journal. Most hospitals and schools have subscriptions to major databases so nurses can access articles at no cost. Connecting patients to evidence-based information is critical to nurses' role in helping them make healthcare decisions.

Not all health-related media on the Internet is as accurate as it should be. When people come to nurses with health information from the Internet, nurses might advise them to look for the logo of the Health on the Net Foundation, an international nonprofit organization that works to verify the reliability of Internet health information. Information on the organization can be found at www.hon.ch. Readers can look for the Health on the Net logo, and click on it at a given Web site to verify that the site is registered with the organization. If so, readers can have some confidence that the Web site at least strives to deliver accurate and evidence-based healthcare information.

Nurses also must take steps to shape the health information individuals see on the Internet and in other media. If the information is not accurate or complete, nurses should try to provide better information by working with the media using the suggestions given previously.

Send Feedback to the Media

It is important that nurses let the media know that they are watching, and that they expect the media to present a fair and accurate account of the profession, especially at a time when nursing is under great stress. Nurses should monitor the media and send feedback. Some examples include sending thanks to the media for accurate or three-dimensional coverage of nursing issues; providing feedback to journalists, individuals, or groups who are responsible for inaccurate or damaging depictions of nurses, as the case study presented earlier illustrates; and mobilizing colleagues to protest poor portrayals of nursing.

Remember that even the entertainment and advertising media have powerful effects on public views of nursing and health, and many people are more likely to engage with health issues that are set in the context of popular entertainment. Many of us are more focused on what's happening on *Grey's Anatomy* than we are on the nightly news, and calling attention to how such entertainment products treat nursing can generate vital public discussion of nursing and its situation.

The media influences healthcare decisions, so nurses have an important responsibility to advocate for more accurate media depictions of nurses and nursing, as well as more accurate and complete messages that will support better decision-making in health care generally. As the Take a Loved One for a Checkup Day campaign shows, changing social perceptions through the media takes time, commitment, and a sustained, cohesive strategy. However, nurses can do it.

References

Ad Council (2013). *Frequently asked questions*. Retrieved from http://www.adcouncil.org/About-Us/Frequently-Asked-Questions

Bohn, R., & Short, J. (2012). Measuring consumer information. *International Journal of Communication, 6*, 986. Retrieved from http://ijoc.org/ojs/index.php/ijoc/article/viewFile/1566/743

Brindley, P. G., & Needham, C. (2009). Positioning prior to endotracheal intubation on a television medical drama: Perhaps life mimics art. *Resuscitation, 80*(5), 604. Retrieved from http://www.resuscitationjournal.com/article/S0300-9572(09)00100-2/abstract

Brodie, M., Foehr, U., Rideout, V., Baer, N., Miller, C., Flournoy, R., et al. (2001). Communicating health information through the entertainment media. *Health Affairs, 20*(1), 192–199. Retrieved from http://content.healthaffairs.org/cgi/reprint/20/1/192

Buresh, B., & Gordon, S. (2006). *From silence to voice: What nurses know and must communicate to the public* (2nd ed.). Ithaca, NY: Cornell University Press.

Center for Nursing Advocacy (2003). *Washington Post highlights center's "ER" campaign*. Retrieved from http://www.truthaboutnursing.org/news/2003/nov/18_washpost.html

Center for Nursing Advocacy (2004a). *Kicking Dr. Phil's ass to the curb*. Retrieved from http://www.truthaboutnursing.org/news/2004/nov/18_dr_phil.html

Center for Nursing Advocacy (2004b). *Killers, tea and sympathy*. Retrieved from http://www.truthaboutnursing.org/news/2004/nov/rd.html

Center for Nursing Advocacy (2005a). *Babynewspaper*. Retrieved from http://www.truthaboutnursing.org/news/2005/dec/04_balt_sun.html

Center for Nursing Advocacy (2005b). *Take a loved one for a checkup day*. Retrieved from http://www.truthaboutnursing.org/news/2005/jul/loved_one.html

Center for Nursing Advocacy (2005c). *As I lay dying*. Retrieved from http://www.truthaboutnursing.org/news/2005/oct/23_boston_globe.html

Center for Nursing Advocacy (2006a). *Family presence and the physician in charge*. Retrieved from http://www.truthaboutnursing.org/news/2006/apr/03_new_yorker.html

Center for Nursing Advocacy (2006b). *CVS pharmacist returns from Matrix; can now download entire nursing curriculum into your brain in four hours!* Retrieved from http://www.truthaboutnursing.org/news/2006/jan/24_cvs.html

Center for Nursing Advocacy (2006c). *Debugging the "electronic nurse."* Retrieved from http://www.truthaboutnursing.org/news/2006/sep/20_electronic_nurse.html

Crockett, R. J., Pruzinsky, T., & Persing, J. A. (2007). The influence of plastic surgery "reality TV" on cosmetic surgery patient expectations and decision making. *Plastic and Reconstructive Surgery, 120*(1), 316–324. Retrieved from http://tinyurl.com/6y97d3

Donnelly, L. (5 August, 2012). Nurses look after 15 patients at a time. *The Telegraph* (London). Retrieved from http://tinyurl.com/cu9b32e

eMarketer.com (2012). *Consumers spending more time with mobile as growth slows for time online*. Retrieved from http://goo.gl/jJwrM

Freed, J. (2006). *Model of the communication cycle: Communication creates reality*. Retrieved http://www.media-visions.com/communication.html

Gallup (2012). *Honesty/ethics in professions*. Retrieved from http://www.gallup.com/poll/1654/honesty-ethics-professions.aspx

Glik, D. C. (2003). *Health communication in popular media formats*. American Public Health Association Annual Meeting presentation. Retrieved from http://www.medscape.com/viewarticle/466709

Henry J. Kaiser Family Foundation (2002). *Survey snapshot: The impact of TV's health content: A case study of ER viewers*. Retrieved from http://www.kff.org/entmedia/3230-index.cfm

Henry J. Kaiser Family Foundation (2003). *Documenting the power of television—a survey of regular E.R. viewers about emergency contraception—summary of findings*. Retrieved from http://www.kff.org/womenshealth/1358-ers.cfm

Henry J. Kaiser Family Foundation (2004). *Entertainment education and health in the United States*. Retrieved from http://www.kff.org/entmedia/7047.cfm

Institute of Medicine (2010). *The future of nursing: Leading change, advancing health*. Retrieved from http://goo.gl/KxxvJ

JWT Communications (2000). *Memo to Nurses for a Healthier Tomorrow coalition members*. Retrieved from http://www.truthaboutnursing.org/research/lit/jwt_memo1.html

Kalisch, B., & Kalisch, P. (n.d.). *The work of Beatrice Kalisch and Philip Kalisch on nursing's public image and the nursing shortage*. Retrieved from http://www.truthaboutnursing.org/research/lit/kalisch_kalisch.html

Kalisch, P. A., & Kalisch, B. J. (1986). A comparative analysis of nurse and physician characters in the entertainment media. *Journal of Advanced Nursing, 11*(2), 179–195.

Kantar Media (2013). *Kantar Media reports U.S. advertising expenditures increased 3 percent in 2012*. Retrieved from http://kantarmediana.com/intelligence/press/us-advertising-expenditures-increased-3-percent-2012

Kelly, J., Fealy, G. M., & Watson, R. (2012). The image of you: Constructing nursing identities in YouTube. *Journal of Advanced Nursing, 68*(8), 1804–1813. Retrieved from http://goo.gl/scnfO

Kwantlen Polytechnic University (n.d.). *If you want to truly understand something, try to change it*. Retrieved from http://www.nursing-informatics.com/N4111/LA1.html

Lewenson, S. B. (1993). *Taking charge: Nursing, suffrage, and feminism in America, 1873–1920*. New York: Garland Press.

Mason, D. J., Leavitt, J. K., & Chafee, M. W. (Eds.) (2011). *Policy and politics in nursing and health care* (6th ed.). St. Louis, MO: Saunders Elsevier.

Neilson, G. R., & Lauder, W. (2008). What do high academic achieving school pupils really think about a career in nursing: Analysis of the narrative from paradigmatic case interviews. *Nurse Education Today, 28*, 680–690. Retrieved from http://www.truthaboutnursing.org/research/lit/neilson_lauder.pdf

Nelson, S., & Gordon, S. (2006). *The complexities of care: Nursing reconsidered*. Ithaca, NY: Cornell University Press.

Norris, P. (2008). The fourth estate. *Driving Democracy*. New York: Cambridge University Press. Retrieved from http://tinyurl.com/a66y2bn

Parker, J. C., & Thorson, E. (2009). *Health communication in the new media landscape*. New York: Springer Publishing Company. Retrieved from http://www.springerpub.com/samples/9780826101228_chapter.pdf

Pew Internet & American Life Project (2011). *The social life of health information, 2011: Summary of findings*. Retrieved from http://goo.gl/XJaJm

Reader's Digest Association (2011) Answers. *Reader's Digest*. Retrieved from www.answers.com/topic/reader-s-digest

Reynolds, K. (1997). *What is the transmission model of interpersonal communication and what is wrong with it?* Student paper from the University of Wales, Aberystwyth. Retrieved from http://www.aber.ac.uk/media/Students/kjr9601.html

Rideout, V. (2008). *Television as a health educator: A case study of Grey's Anatomy*. Kaiser Family Foundation. Retrieved from http://www.kff.org/entmedia/7803.cfm

Rimal, R. N., & Lapinski, M. K. (2009). Why health communication is important in public health. *Bulletin of the World Health Organization, 87*, 247. Retrieved from http://goo.gl/2oDTI

Sapatkin, D. (31 July, 2012). Penn study examines link between nurse burnout, care. *Philadelphia Inquirer*. Retrieved from http://goo.gl/VOyBI

Stringer, H. (2012). *Johnson & Johnson Campaign for Nursing's Future turns 10*. Retrieved from http://goo.gl/RmCAm

Summers, S., & Summers, H. J. (2010). *Saving lives: Why the media's portrayal of nurses puts us all at risk*. New York: Kaplan Publishing.

The Truth About Nursing (2009). *Take the blue pill*. Retrieved from http://www.truthaboutnursing.org/news/2009/jul/06_jackie.html#presence

The Truth About Nursing (2010). *Mercy reviews*. Retrieved from http://www.truthaboutnursing.org/media/tv/mercy.html

The Truth About Nursing (2011a). *HawthoRNe reviews*. Retrieved from http://www.truthaboutnursing.org/media/tv/hawthorne.html

The Truth About Nursing (2011b). *Johnson & Johnson nurse television commercials*. Retrieved from http://www.truthaboutnursing.org/media/commercials/jnj.html

The Truth About Nursing (2011c). *That leg brace graduated first in its nursing school class!* Retrieved from http://www.truthaboutnursing.org/news/2011/nov/robots.html

The Truth About Nursing (2011d). *Do physicians deliver better care than advanced practice registered nurses?* Retrieved from http://www.truthaboutnursing.org/faq/aprn_md.html

The Truth About Nursing (2012a). *Why aren't you more excited that public opinion polls often put nurses at the top of the list of "most trusted" and "most ethical" professions?*

Retrieved from http://www.truthaboutnursing.org/faq/most_trusted.html

The Truth About Nursing (2012b). *The Truth About Nursing awards rank best and worst media portrayals of nursing*. Retrieved from http://www.truthaboutnursing.org/press/awards/

The Truth About Nursing (2012c). *Call the Midwife episode reviews*. Retrieved from http://www.truthaboutnursing.org/media/tv/call_the_midwife.html

The Truth About Nursing (2012d). *Nurse Jackie episode reviews*. Retrieved from http://www.truthaboutnursing.org/media/tv/nurse_jackie.html

The Truth About Nursing (2013). *Are you sure nurses are autonomous? Based on what I've seen, it sure looks like physicians are calling the shots*. Retrieved from http://www.truthaboutnursing.org/faq/autonomy.html

Turow, J., & Gans, R. (2002). *As seen on TV: Health policy issues in TV's medical dramas*. Report to the Henry J. Kaiser Family Foundation, p. 1. Retrieved from http://www.kff.org/entmedia/3231-index.cfm

U.S. Department of Health and Human Services, Health Resources and Service Administration (2010). *The registered nurse population: Initial findings from the 2008 national sample survey of registered nurses*. Retrieved from http://goo.gl/rLmWK

U.S. Department of Health and Human Services Press Office (2004). *HHS Secretary Tommy G. Thompson launches third annual "Take a loved one to the doctor day."* Retrieved from http://archive.hhs.gov/news/press/2004pres/20040712.html

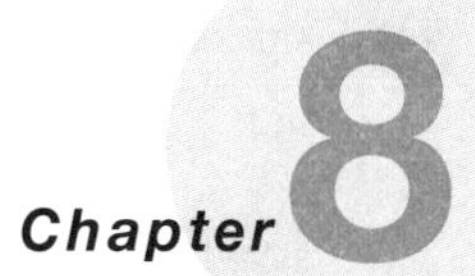

Chapter 8

Working Together: Shared Decision-Making

Marie Truglio-Londrigan and

Cheryl Barnes

The complexities of the U.S. healthcare system warrant an approach to clinical practice, education, and research that is inclusive of all disciplines and the populations that these disciplines serve. Individual practitioners, educators, and researchers find themselves making clinical decisions at the point of service throughout their daily practice. These same practitioners also may find that working together in groups is essential to their practice as they attempt to meet the complex challenges that are an ever-increasing reality. These challenges include the rise of mental health issues and chronic illnesses, violence, infectious diseases, weak public health infrastructure, disaster management, threats of terrorism, the rapid expansion of technology, fragmented health care, an aging population, and the realities of a limited pool of resources including financial and people power as evidenced by a continual struggle to maintain a sustainable nursing workforce. Bruce and McKane (2000) discuss the importance of communities, health practitioners, and academicians working together to meet these challenges. Working together in groups may take place in a wide variety of forums. Two such examples include groups of individuals who work together as in interdisciplinary teams in healthcare organizations or groups of organizations who work together in formal or informal coalitions. This coming *together* to work *together* leads to the notion of making decisions *together*. Working together in groups, therefore, allows individuals or organizations to come together to work toward a goal and ultimately achieve their vision via shared decision-making.

The purpose of this chapter is twofold. The first part of this chapter focuses on group work in teams, specifically an interdisciplinary team as it operates in a healthcare organization. It describes how this interdisciplinary team functions and makes shared decisions. The second part of the chapter explores the development of partnerships within coalitions. Specifically, the chapter provides a presentation of an informal coalition in a community setting with a highlight on their shared decision-making process. Group work and the inherent process of the group that leads to shared decision-making is an important competency for nurses to learn and use in any practice environment.

Group Work and Shared Decision-Making on an Interdisciplinary Team

The Institute of Medicine (IOM) report, *To Err Is Human: Building a Safer Health System* (Kohn, Corrigan, & Donaldson, 2000), outlined the toll that medical errors take every year on individuals, families, communities, organizations, and the healthcare system in general. In response to this, the IOM produced *Crossing the Quality Chasm: A New Health System for the 21st Century* (Committee on Quality of Health Care in America, 2001). This report outlined the need for a "sweeping redesign" (p. 2). An important component of this redesign concerned the preparation of the healthcare workforce in a way that facilitated an interdisciplinary focus. This focus was further exemplified in *Health Professions Education: A Bridge to Quality* (Greiner & Knebel, 2003). Documented within this report is a vision of health professions education that includes five competencies: patient-centered care, interdisciplinary teams, evidence-based practice, quality improvement, and informatics. This work was further developed by the Quality and Safety Education for Nurses (QSEN) project. Based on the previous works noted, QSEN participants developed quality and safety competencies for nursing. These competencies include patient-centered care, teamwork and collaboration, evidence-based practice, quality improvement, safety, and informatics (Cronenwett et al., 2007). The Interprofessional Education Collaborative (IPEC) (2011) further examined, developed, and defined the Interprofessional Collaborative Practice Competency Domains as values/ethics for interprofessional practice, roles/responsibilities, interprofessional communication, teams, and teamwork (p. 16).

It is clear that there has been an enhanced interest in the notion of group work and the outcomes resulting from the decisions of the group, more specifically, interdisciplinary teams and the outcomes of these collaborative endeavors to build a "safer and better patient-centered and community/population oriented U.S. health care system" (IPEC, 2011, p. 3). Nurses do have a significant role in this redesign, given our vast numbers and the ability of nurses to practice in a multitude of areas where we are at the pinnacle point of service. To this end, the IOM report titled *The Future of Nursing: Leading Change, Advancing Health* (Committee on the Robert Wood Johnson Foundation, 2011) outlined four key messages. One of these messages points to the need for nurses to be full partners with physicians and other healthcare professionals. In addition to these four key messages were recommendations, one of which clearly articulated the need for nurses to lead collaborative initiatives with physicians and other members of the healthcare team. It is clear what we do is important, but in this redesign it is also clear that how we do it, focusing on collaboration and working together in interdisciplinary teams where decision-making as a competency is essential for the success of the group, is equally as important (IPEC, 2011).

The notion of group work in a team has been present in the literature for many decades. For instance, the IOM (1972) published a report titled *Educating for the Health Team* that highlighted the discussions that took place at the national level on the subject of interdisciplinary education and to answer questions pertaining to interdisciplinary teams. Today in our healthcare environment the notion of teams has never been more important and is highly visible. A team has been noted to be a group of people (Finkelman & Kenner, 2010). An interdisciplinary team, therefore, is also a group of individuals. More specifically the interdisciplinary team is:

> . . . composed of members from different professions and occupations with varied and specialized knowledge, skills, and methods. The team members integrate their observations, bodies of expertise, and spheres of decision making to coordinate, collaborate, and communicate with one another in order to optimize care for a patient or group of patients. (Greiner & Knebel, 2003, p. 54)

The essence of this interdisciplinary team is how it works together in an integrated manner, as one, toward the achievement of a team-specified goal. As such, we suggest that working together in a team does not just happen. The team and the work of the team are a collective and collaborative effort that the members, as well as the organization that the team members work for, must work to achieve. In order to do this successfully there must be trust and respect. Porter-O'Grady and Malloch (2011) noted that trust among members, group identity, and a sense of group efficacy are necessary if a team is to be fully engaged. This engagement of each member of the team is essential because it facilitates the "... interconnectedness of members and acknowledge[s] the unique contributions of each to the delivery of services ... to make substantial contributions to the achievements of organizational goals" (p. 340). Porter-O'Grady and Malloch (2011) also suggest that emotional competence of all team members is an important precursor to successful teamwork. The individual who is emotionally competent exhibits "... a high regard for colleagues and subordinates, an understanding of basic motivations as well as basic justice, a willingness to take responsibility, a willingness to correct faulty situations, and a willingness to take positive, quick, and aggressive action when indicated" (p. 321). The selection of team members who display the qualities of emotional competence and/or the potential for emotional competence, therefore, may facilitate the working of the team. It also suggests that education, mentoring, nurturing, and coaching of the team, in this regard, may prove to be important strategies to be developed that may ultimately both facilitate and enhance the team's work. Teams in which each member demonstrates emotional competence strive to listen to and understand each member's perspectives. Herein is the essence of "team work." Too often when individuals work together, listening does not occur. Individuals hear their own voice and do not hear the voices of the many. For teams to be truly functioning as a team there needs to be an effort to listen to the individual so that the collective may be heard with an eye on the ultimate goal.

The establishment of teams is complex, and therefore in any healthcare organization the development of team members and teams takes time, education, and reflective thought. There are many models that may be applied as guides to the development and initiation of a team. An example of a complex system designed to assist healthcare organizations in their successful implementation of teams is the TeamSTEPPS project. TeamSTEPPS is a teamwork system designed for healthcare professionals. It is:

- A solution to improving patient safety.
- An evidence-based teamwork system to improve communication and teamwork skills.
- A source for ready-to-use materials and a training curriculum to integrate teamwork principles.
- Based in more than 20 years of research and lessons from the application of teamwork.
- Developed by Department of Defense's Patient Safety Program in collaboration with the Agency for Healthcare Research and

> Quality. (U.S. Department of Health and Human Services, Agency for Healthcare Research and Quality, n.d., para 1)

The U.S. Department of Health and Human Services, Agency for Healthcare Research and Quality TeamSTEPPS Web site (http://teamstepps.ahrq.gov) presents the reader with a vast offering of information, tools, materials, assessments, training, educational materials, supportive networking, stories of implementation projects, and training events such as conferences to assist any professional or organization in their team initiation efforts. An example of effective teamwork in an acute care setting may be viewed in the following case study.

Case Study

An exemplar that demonstrates effective interdisciplinary teamwork and decision-making involved a 38-year-old with end-stage ovarian cancer. Mrs. M was a married mother of two girls ages 8 and 11 years. Mrs. M had multiple health issues related to her recurrent cancer and was admitted to the hospital with a small bowel obstruction for which she had a drainage percutaneous endoscopic gastrostomy tube placed. In addition she had bilateral percutaneous nephrostomies placed due to bilateral hydronephrosis caused by tumor growth around her ureters. With the progression of her disease, Mrs. M and her husband decided on no further active treatment for her cancer and opted to be made DNR and to be discharged home with home hospice. With the complexity of the situation involving alteration in nutrition, functioning, body image, pain management, and role function as a mother and wife, collaboration among the interdisciplinary team members was necessary to achieve this outcome.

The team consisted of the primary nurse, nurse case manager, social worker, pharmacist, nurse practitioner, primary medical doctor, psychiatry, pain and palliative team, rehab team, dietician, and the patient and her family. Effective teamwork was essential in developing a plan of care that was mutually satisfying to the patient, caregivers, and providers. The goal of the team was to promote individualized, culturally congruent discharge plans for the patient by empowering the patient, significant others, and caregivers through reflection, information sharing, consensus building, and identification of a common purpose, keeping the focus on the patient. Team members were committed to teaching each other, learning from each other, and working across boundaries to plan and provide integrated services to the patient. In the end, the intended outcome of a safe and timely discharge of the patient through improved information flow and effective interventions with optimum patient, provider, and family satisfaction was achieved.

In this case study the group work of the interdisciplinary team is clearly in evidence. It is also evident that there is a real sharing between and among all members of the team as information is presented, described, and shared so that ultimately there is a shared decision. The shared decisions of the particular team, in this case study, is an exemplar of a model of shared decision-making presented by Légaré, Stacey, Briére et al., (2011) and (Légaré, Stacey, Pouliot et al., 2011). These authors presented a model of shared decision-making that moves beyond the traditional dyad model of healthcare provider and patient to a model that is representative of the interprofessional team and patient known as the Interprofessional Shared Decision-Making model (IP-SDM). The notion of shared decision-making in the context of teams is also discussed by Truglio-Londrigan (2013) in her qualitative work entitled *Shared Decision-Making in Home-Care from the Nurse's Perspective: Sitting at the Kitchen Table*. In this qualitative inquiry several themes emerged. One theme *The Village and Shared Decision-Making* identifies how shared decision-making does not necessarily exist between the healthcare provider and the patient alone but a much more expansive view of practice needs to be considered that includes groups of individuals, for example, in the model of a team.

Group Work and Shared Decision-Making in a Coalition Partnership Model

Some individuals propose that when working together in groups the decision-making process yields better decisions, because of the collective input into the process (Yoder-Wise, 2003). Groups provide for varied input because of the involvement of multiple members and generate a greater commitment (Sullivan & Decker, 2005). Groups may take many forms and follow many different models. For the purpose of this part of the chapter, however, the work of the group will be discussed in relation to a group of organizations or agencies that are working together in a coalition partnership model.

A coalition is two or more organizations coming together that join forces and share resources so that a shared concern is challenged and resolved (Sullivan, 1998). Furthermore, a coalition "promotes and develops alliances among organizations or constituencies for a common purpose. It builds linkages, solves problems, and/or enhances local leadership to address health concerns" (Keller, Strohschein, & Briske, 2008, p. 204). Because of the linkages and the resulting collaboration, resources are frequently shared, thereby enhancing capitol, resulting in maximization of outcomes (Wald, 2013). More specifically Wald (2013) stated "Because a range of local interests is represented and brought together, forming a coalition can build a powerful base of key individuals or organizations that can work to influence social change of a mutual concern" (p. 306). The strengthening of the social fabric of a community is also seen as an outcome (Butterfoss, Goodman, & Wandersman, 1993). According to the Center for Prevention Research and Development (2006), coalitions broaden

> . . . the mission of member organizations and develop more comprehensive strategies, develop wider public support for issues/actions; increase influence of community institutions over community policies and practices; minimize duplication of services; develop more financial and human resources; increase participation from diverse sectors and constituencies; exploit resources in changing environments; and increase accountability. (p. 2)

There are many types of coalitions noted in the literature. Coalitions may be developed as a permanent measure or to achieve temporary goals. In addition, coalitions may be illustrative of a grassroots effort developed and organized from the bottom up by volunteers, professionally organized, or community-based initiated by both professionals and individuals within a community (Feighery & Rogers, 1990; Wald, 2013). The significance of a coalition is noted when one considers the "...complex, multi-layered problems that require sophisticated solutions at the community level. Coalitions by themselves are not a prevention strategy, but a means whereby a community can organize, plan, and deliver multi-level and multi-faceted prevention programs, policies and practices" (Center for Prevention Research and Development, 2006, p. 3).

Community Coalition Action Theory

From the brief review of the literature pertaining to coalitions and the partnerships inherent within these coalitions it is evident that the structure and processes that take place throughout the organizational framework of coalitions are indeed complex. To facilitate a greater understanding, Butterfoss and Kegler (2009) presented the Community Coalition Action Theory (CCAT).

The authors of this model speak to specific stages in the creation and maintenance of a coalition. These stages include formation, maintenance, and institutionalization. The stages are cyclical in nature, not linear (Butterfoss & Kegler, 2009; Butterfoss, 2007); therefore, they more accurately represent the work of a coalition as new initiatives are born and older initiatives are evaluated, leading to the development and implementation of new strategies based on new data and best practice. Other constructs of the CCAT include: community context, lead agency/convening group, coalition membership, processes, leadership and staffing, structures, member engagement and pooled resources, assessment and planning, implementation of strategies, community change outcomes, health/social outcomes, and community capacity (Butterfoss & Kegler, 2009; Butterfoss, 2007).

To delve into the workings of the coalition using this model is beyond the scope of this chapter. A brief summation, however, is in order. First and foremost, there may be a pressing need in the community along with other community contextual factors. The lead organization, such as a state department of health, may act as a convener or a broker of other organizations. The lead organization may host an initial meeting or provide initial support in some way. The original core group ultimately expands, providing a larger, more diverse representation of the community including formal organizations, public groups, private companies, and key individuals in the community who may have an expressed interest in participating. These community organizations may share similar ideas, values, and beliefs pertaining to the identified issue and may have a desire to work with the lead organization. Thus, the early formulation stage of the coalition is noted. The structures and processes of the coalition are soon formalized including the development of the vision and the mission statement. As the coalition continues to work, attention must be given to the development of a formal structure that is flat, not hierarchical, which facilitates shared decision-making (Osmond, n.d.). As the members of the coalition work together there is a pooling of member resources, thereby facilitating assessment, researching of best practice strategies, planning, implementation of best practice strategies, and evaluation. Throughout this process attention is given to communication, collaboration, shared work, shared problem solving, and shared goal setting, all of which are facilitated via shared decision-making that is supported by trust over time.

What Is Needed for a Successful Coalition?

What was described in the previous section represents a structure and process strategy for encouraging problem solving, particularly in community settings (Kaye & Wolff, 2002). Those organizations that come together to work together in a collaborative way. This collaboration is defined as "a dynamic transforming process of creating a power sharing partnership for pervasive application in health care practice, education, research, and organizational settings for the purposeful attention to needs and problems in order to achieve likely successful outcomes . . ." (Sullivan, 1998, p. 6).

Reflecting on the definition of coalitions just given, several characteristics clearly are evident. These include a dynamic transforming process, power-sharing partnerships, attention to needs and problems, and successful outcomes. Inherent in these characteristics are the important concepts of relationships, trust, and group work where the decision-making is shared. In order for there to be a power-sharing partnership, some type of relationship must be evident. Initially, the partnership is held together because of the vision that may have brought the group together. For example, a community coalition may consist of several health, educational, and social organizations of a local town wanting to plan and build a skate park for its young residents. This skate park may be used by skateboarders and in-liners, who are usually a particular aggregate of the preteen and teen population in a given community. Early in the development of the coalition, the partnership and the relationship among all of the organizations is held together by their vision. In this case, the vision is the need for a safe environment for the community's young residents so that they may practice their sport in a safe manner.

The relationships that take form in the development of the coalition reflect a complex network of connections that sets the stage for the development of trust. As the coalition works together over time, affirming their relationship, trust is established and strengthened. With this relationship building, connection, and the development of trust, communication takes place throughout. Kang (1997) notes that trusting relationships facilitate efficiency and fidelity in communication and the diffusion of information. Similarly, Cartwright and Limandri (1997) note that trust is essential for open expression of views and opinions. The building of a trusting relationship within the partnerships of the coalition facilitates the coalition's ability to communicate and share in the decision-making process together. Trust, therefore, facilitates a climate of openness that aids the work of the coalition (Porter-O'Grady & Malloch, 2011). These authors further stressed the importance of trust when they clarified "Three conditions—trust among members, a sense of group identity, and a sense of group efficacy—are essential to effectiveness" (Porter-O'Grady & Malloch, 2011, p. 340). This trust is essential because without it, the coalition will not be a success. The primary reason for an unsuccessful ending is the inability of the coalition to share not only in the work, but also in the decision-making so necessary for a coalition's survival. Foster-Fishman, Berkowitz, Lounsbury, Jacobson, and Allen (2001) carried out a qualitative analysis of 80 articles, chapters, and practitioners' guides focusing on coalition functioning in an attempt to identify core competencies and processes necessary for coalition success and the building of this capacity. These were noted to be the following (Foster-Fishman et al., 2001):

- *Member capacity:* This includes skills and knowledge needed by coalition members so that they may work collaboratively together, create programs and build an effective and strong infrastructure, and develop and sustain motivational attitudes about the coalition and the inherent collaborative efforts regarding the targeted issue and program, all while maintaining positive attitudes about other stakeholders and self.
- *Relational capacity:* This includes developing a shared vision, promoting power sharing and participatory decision-making, and creating a positive working environment that values diversity of interests and views.
- *Organizational capacity:* This includes leadership and developing effective processes and procedures along with effective forms of communication and the assurance of internal and external resources.
- *Programmatic capacity:* This includes development of goals, with strategies based in best practice to achieve those stated goals.

All of these are essential for a successful coalition, and time must be devoted to the development of strategies to ensure the building of these various capacities. One area of particular importance for this chapter is the area of shared decision-making and what is meant by the group sharing in the discussion and decision-making process within these coalitions.

Working Together Towards Shared Decision-Making: The Common Good

The overriding vision of the coalition serves as the driving force. The key term here is *overriding*. In other words, when the individual members of the coalition make formal or informal agreements to come together with the expressed purpose of working toward the vision, there is a common ground that has been established for the achievement of the common good. This shared vision leads to a shared mission and goals. It is the idea of working together for the common good that keeps the coalition vital as the partners share in the work and decision-making. The shared vision is the driving force, the engine, that supports the activities of the coalition including shared work, shared problem solving, shared responsibility, shared goal setting, and shared planning, throughout which shared group decision-making takes place (Sullivan, 1998). Shared vision and mission are essential not only for the work of the coalition, but also for the creation of a "community change" that will be sustained (Cramer, Atwood, & Stoner, 2006, p. 71). A visual representation of this is noted in **Figure 8-1**. This model is similar to the model of decision-making being put forth in this text. Every step

Figure 8-1

Visual representation of group decision-making.

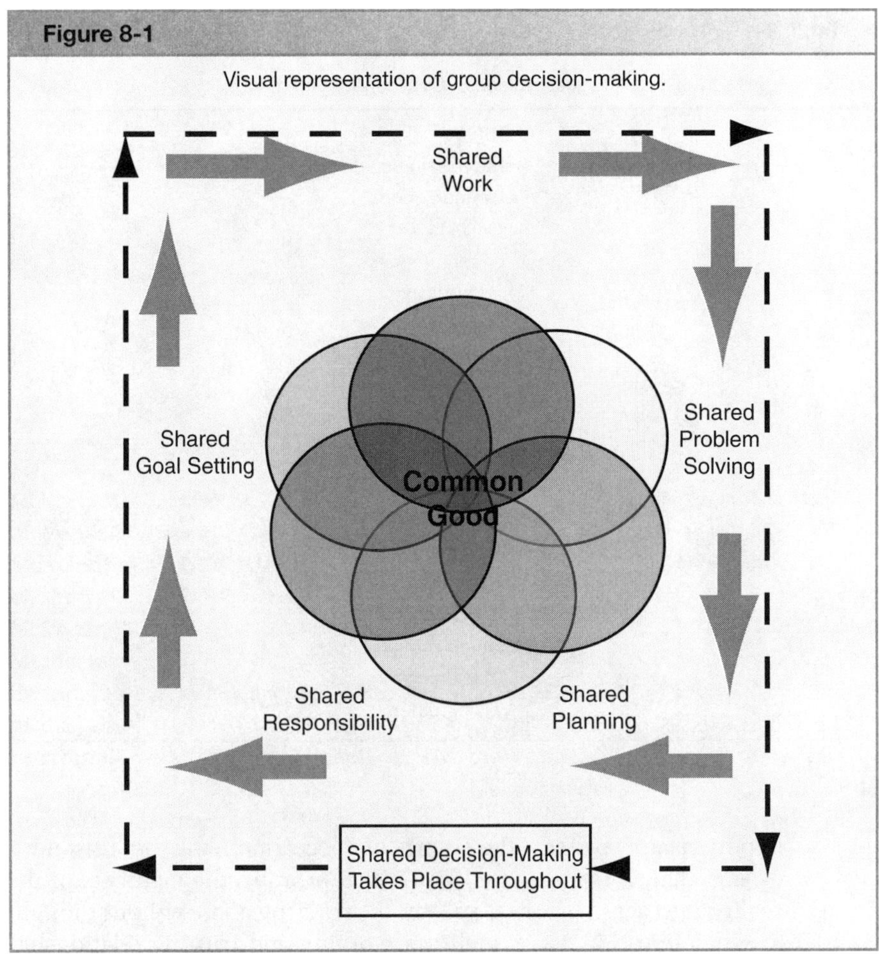

in the process of coalition development and in the coalition's work toward the achievement of the vision or the mission and goals of this model is enacted because of the coalition's ability to share in the work, at every level for the common good.

Shared Values and Collective Action for the Common Good

There are many shared values and actions (**Table 8-1**) that support a coalition's work and facilitate the decision-making process. The overriding vision presented earlier is the core from which the mission and goals are developed. Together, the shared vision, mission, and goals are

Table 8-1

Shared Values of Coalition Members
Shared vision
Shared mission/goal
Common good
Collectivism
Other-centeredness
Broad participation
Inclusiveness
Respect
Time
Self-reflection
Sharing
Power with
Being present
Being attentive
Intention
Collegiality
Communication
Listening
Valuing others

important and represent the essence of the coalition, the very reason for its existence. It is this shared vision that prompts the members of the coalition to act in a collective way, to work together without thought to self-interest. It is a model of a working and trusting relationship in which the common good is given precedence over the interests of the individual organizations involved. This illustrates another value of equal importance, which is that the members of a coalition need to be other-centered for the support and facilitation of the common good.

In order for there to be a sharing in the decision-making process among all members of a coalition, the decision-making process must permit "broad participation in determining the course of the coalition" (Kaye & Wolff, 2002, p. 33). The primary concern is the vision of the entire coalition; therefore, the voices of all of the members of the coalition must be heard and valued. In this type of decision-making, there is a kind of collectivism in which all of the organizations involved share in the work—including the planning, task accomplishments, implementation of strategies, and evaluation of outcomes—in a way that exemplifies inclusiveness (Woehrle, 2003). A coalition is nonhierarchical. There is no "power over" in a coalition, only "power with" as the members of the coalition exemplify the values of sharing and inclusiveness for the common good. This requires equal empowerment of all members of a coalition in order for the entity to communicate and work together. Any opposition to this broad participation and inclusiveness inhibits the working of the coalition. Working with groups that also may include consumers is challenging and there always is the possibility for hierarchical relationships, which may result in decisions that are not representative of the view of the entire group (Allen, Dyas, & Jones, 2004). This, however, violates the spirit of a coalition.

This highlights yet another value essential to the entire collective process: the value of shared communication and the respect for the time necessary for this shared communication to take place. The communication exchange that takes place among all organizational members of the coalition must be considered and must demonstrate the inclusiveness discussed earlier to engage all members' perspectives: "Exclusion generates 'we–they' dynamic; . . . What is needed is a pluralistic process . . ." (Michaels, 2002, p. 2). Part of this time is needed for self-reflection. The communication necessary for the entire sharing process including shared decision-making is complex. Greitemeyer, Schulz-Hardt, Brodbeck, and Frey (2006) identify that making decisions in organizations and in life where there are groups as players in the decision-making process requires more time and effort among the people involved. Members of the coalition must consciously be present, attentive, and listen with intention in every respect. Michaels (2002) speaks to this same issue and notes that through the ". . . practice of listening, intentional speaking, and conscious self-monitoring . . ." (p. 1), the purpose of the group will be realized. There is no room for an atmosphere of competition, only collegiality and working together for the common good. Self-reflection enables members of the coalition to become involved in moments of self-checking, asking questions such as: How do I feel about what is happening? Can I support what is happening? Do I feel listened to? Do I feel that what I have to say is valued? Is the coalition taking on a task that is congruent with the original vision, mission, and goals? Is any one member of the coalition attempting to usurp power? Answers to these questions may give clues to how one feels about the progress and process of the coalition and how one is responding or reacting to others in the coalition at any given moment in time, thus avoiding conflict.

Why Consensus?

As previously stated individuals may work together in groups representing teams and organizations that partner and work together may be illustrative of coalitions. In both cases the groups share in the work, discussions, and the decisions representing shared decision-making. An example of this sharing in decisions is consensus. Consensus is nonhierarchical; instead, decisions are made through a collective and participatory approach. Woehrle (2003) notes that "consensus is that 'general agreement' is reached" (p. 15) and the process that unfolds in the group that facilitates this "general agreement." This process illustrates "harmony, cooperation, sympathy, and group solidarity. . . . It does require people willing to find common ground in principle and practical solutions that everyone can live with" (Senge et al., 1999, pp. 378–379). There is no vote whereby the majority "wins" and the minority "loses"; rather, the group process is such that everyone has the opportunity to participate, share, and contribute and the outcome is a decision that everyone believes they can live with (Woehrle, 2003). Groups that make decisions using the majority rule may only "partially achieve the goals of quality and acceptance" (Yoder-Wise, 2003, p. 82) in reference to both the decision being made and the members of the coalition. Woehrle (2003) describes how in the consensus process, it is better to hold off on a decision than to take a vote that excludes individuals: "The balancing factor in consensus is that participants hold the responsibility to 'step aside' if their concerns are not pressing enough to merit blocking the unity of the group" (p. 16). How the group accomplishes this is through the provision of time for dialogue. With time and the dialogue that unfolds, coalition members begin to see and understand what other coalition members may be speaking about, and in time these thoughts and ideas become integrated into their own. This idea is synonymous with Gadamer's (1976) concept of the language of conversation that provides the medium for understanding as individuals use language to express themselves and listen. The outcome is consensus. As Woehrle (2003) described this experience: ". . . time is spent on the process of persuasion" (p. 4).

Techniques and Tools for Consensus

This consensus process is not easy. The one overriding factor that is important throughout the process is that the coalition holds true to the value of the common good and the vision at hand. This is what spurs the coalition members to continue with the discussion and decision-making process until consensus is reached. Members of the coalition may use certain techniques and tools to facilitate the brainstorming of ideas thus contributing to the communication and the generation of alternative ideas. First and foremost, the members of the coalition need to understand group process and consensus. Living in a culture where competition and winning is a primary value means time must be dedicated to education so coalition members come to understand what consensus is and how to work together. Exercises on communication and listening skills may be necessary. Similarly, education on conduct within the group also is essential, particularly the roles inherent in the group.

Consensus does not mean that people just get together and speak without thought to process. In fact, the process is facilitated by the members in the group, who all assume certain roles and responsibilities. AIDS Coalition to Unleash Power (2006) identifies several roles key to the process of consensus building including facilitator, vibes-watcher, and recorder. Huber (2006) identifies the facilitator as the one who "conducts the meeting, ensuring that everyone has the opportunity to speak, maintains the focus of the meeting, and controls the problem participants" (p. 577). The facilitator may be the individual(s) who represents the lead organization of the coalition. This individual facilitates the process with agenda setting, gets all participants involved in the communication and in the work of the coalition, defines and redefines the vision, and works with all members of the coalition to brainstorm when it comes to making decisions or identifying alternative approaches and solutions to problem solving (Conflict Research Consortium, 1998). This brainstorming is just one technique, among many, that may be used to create an environment in which ideas are freely expressed without critique. The goal is to stimulate as many ideas as possible (Yoder-Wise, 2003). Part of the facilitator's role when generating alternatives is to work with the members of the coalition as they collectively evaluate costs and benefits as well as barriers to implementation of the alternatives discussed (Conflict Research Consortium, 1998).

In a given situation where a particular decision must be made, the facilitator, after a period of time brainstorming, assists the group in narrowing down the alternatives to one approach in the form of a proposal. It is the facilitator's responsibility to ensure that all individuals were given the time to express their own ideas and beliefs. Once the final proposal is noted and there appear to be no new ideas being generated for that proposal, the facilitator may ask if there are any objections to its implementation (AIDS Coalition to Unleash Power, 2006). If after a period of silence there are no objections, then consensus is reached. Note how this entire process is one of shared participation and a sharing in the decision. If there are members of the coalition who cannot support the proposal, then they may express their objection. Some members of the coalition may express their objection, yet indicate that they will still abide by the proposal in the interest of the vision of the coalition. Other members of the coalition may not be able to support the proposal and may not be able to abide by the proposal on any level. In this event, the members of the coalition note this and there is a reaffirming of the vision and a return to the process.

Two other roles, vibes-watcher and recorder, are critical to the consensus process. The *vibes-watcher* is a member of the coalition who works side by side with the facilitator. This individual assists the facilitator as they watch the workings of the group and comments on what he or she observes in terms of individual participation, communication patterns within the group, and how individuals within the group are relating—or not—to one another. The *recorder* is the individual who documents the discussions and manages the agenda and time. This role is important because the individual keeps a record of the discussion for archival purposes and for the instances when the group needs to review what discussions have been held in the past (AIDS Coalition to Unleash Power, 2006).

Outcomes of Consensus

According to Yoder-Wise (2003), the outcomes that occur as a result of engaging in consensus are evident because of the different individuals and organizations involved: ". . . when individuals with different knowledge, skills, and resources collaborate to solve a problem or make a decision, the likelihood of a quality outcome is increased" (p. 82). The inclusiveness of the group and the participation among all members of the coalition creates an environment rich with diversity of opinion. These varying opinions that are brought to the group are born out of individually rich experiences and histories. This atmosphere serves to create an environment of growth, commitment, and innovation (Mansbridge, 2003). It makes sense, therefore, that in situations where individuals are directly involved in a coalition driven by consensus—where sharing has taken place throughout the entire process—that there is an enhanced likelihood that decisions and the acceptance of these decisions are increased because all parties have shared in the process. Other advantages include an increase in unity, commitment, innovation, and trust (Mansbridge, 2003).

Nurses work with others in every practice arena and have done so historically as well. An understanding of decision-making that involves others, such as in teams and coalitions, can only serve to enhance and enrich nursing practice and quality as well as safety outcomes. In addition, the outcome of a practice that applies and supports this decision-making process is solutions that are sustainable over time. An example of this informal coalition shared decision-making process is noted in the following case study.

Case Study

In the northeastern United States there is a town located not far from a major city. One spring, the local elementary school nurse heard the students in the elementary school complaining about the town police. Their complaint centered around one particular topic. They were skateboarders and in-line skaters with no place to practice their sport. As a result, these young teens found themselves grinding curbs and handrails anywhere possible. (*Grinding* means the teens use their skateboards on sidewalks, curbs, and staircase railings.) More often than not, these curbs and handrails were on town property, on private property, or in parking lots. The elementary school nurse in the town spoke to the young teens and noted that the conflict that was arising centered on the fact that the police were only trying to protect these young teens and other people in the town who found themselves accosted by the fast-moving action of these young individuals practicing their sport.

The elementary school nurse was a resident of the town and decided to observe these young teens performing their sport. What the school nurse found was that indeed the practice of a much-loved sport was in evidence. With each trick on the skateboard came "whoops and hollers" from the group, supporting one another to "keep going" or to "keep trying." The school nurse also noted that most, if not all, of the young teens were not wearing protective gear and many found themselves in the direct line of oncoming traffic. In fact, the school nurse noted that there had been a recent death in another town as a young teen skateboarded in a major parking lot. As a school nurse, health promotion and protection from injury was always in the forefront of practice. This school nurse gathered the young teens into her office and made a recommendation: "Why don't you go to the town hall and speak with the head of the recreation department? Maybe, just maybe, the town would be willing to work to build you a park." At the beginning, the young teens looked at the nurse with disbelief and asked: "How could this be? Would someone actually be willing to listen to us?"

After this initial meeting with the school nurse, the students, along with their parents, went to the town hall to speak with the director of the department of recreation. The director was willing to listen; however, he wanted evidence that there was a need for a special park, and he wanted to see that other individuals and organizations supported such an idea. From this second meeting, it was clear to the young teens and their families that if their vision—a place to practice their sport in a safe environment—was to become a reality, they needed to contact other organizations. Parents and the young teens put their heads together and came up with a list. The school system, the police department, town board leaders, the department of recreation, the chamber of commerce, a local medical group, and the hospital were all organizations or agencies that had an interest in this particular issue.

The parents and young teens called a third meeting that included all of the listed organizations. All of the organizations displayed an interest and all wanted to work together to build a skate park for this population; thus, an informal coalition was developed. Some were primarily interested in getting "the kids off of the streets" and some were interested in "protecting the young teens from injury."

The various constituents that came together shared an overriding vision, which was to build a skate park for this particular population of young teens. The lead organization was the department of recreation. This department assumed responsibility for any and all town recreation activities. An assessment of such activities revealed that indeed there were many local recreational activities—soccer, swimming, basketball, football, golf, disk golf, hockey, bowling, and tennis, just to name a few—but nothing to support the individuals who practiced skateboarding. Although there was plenty of anecdotal evidence that suggested this to be an unsafe sport if practiced outside of a designated area, there was no objective data such as number of fractures in the emergency room due to skateboarding accidents as a result of not wearing protective gear. The lead agency noted that although this would be great evidence, they were willing to support the skateboard park with the anecdotal evidence if there were enough teens who would be using the park, and if funding could be found to support this type of park.

All the members of this informal coalition took on separate distinct roles, yet each coalition member was integral to the achievement of the vision. The recreation department was the lead organization and responsible for ensuring that communication was sustained among all members. The facilitator of the meetings, the director of the recreation department, ensured that all members of the coalition—especially the young teens—had a say in the discussion and that all members were listened to. Meetings were held at times convenient to everyone.

During these meetings, the vision of the skateboard park remained at the forefront with the discussions centered on how to realize that vision. Several times during the planning process, the members of the coalition went to town meetings to keep the town board advised as to the process. The chamber of commerce was involved so that the town businesses were kept in the loop about the status of the park because of their hope that these young teens would stop practicing in front of their stores. This involvement also was important because the business members in town also would be influential with fundraising throughout efforts. The hospital and the medical group provided the information pertaining to the need for such a park, with particular emphasis on the health promotion and protection of this young population of teens. The school system, local elementary school nurse, and town police supported the students in their planning and in the generation of ideas for fundraising along with the parents. The parents and teens were responsible for heading up the fundraising efforts as well as the planning and building of the park. The key here was the young teens actively engaging in the planning of the park design so that they would have a hand in the selection of the pipes and ramps that they found most useful for practicing their sport.

Key decisions made by the coalition included the need for the park, the location of the park, the equipment in the park, how to raise money for the park, how to build the park, the monitoring of the park once built, rules of conduct in the park, and fees to use the park.

As with any coalition, all members' ideas were critical to the success of the vision. In this case study, shared decision-making using consensus was in evidence throughout. For example, when looking for an appropriate site to build the park, all members of the coalition assessed every available free space within the town. Given that there was not a tremendous amount of unused space, this presented only three options. The coalition members engaged in discussion about these three spaces under the guidance of the director of the department of recreation. Ultimately, all members respected the others and listened to alternative solutions. In the end, the proposal for one particular site was met with agreement by all members of the coalition. In the final analysis, the skateboard park was built and the use of the park by the young teens has been in strong evidence.

Conclusion

In today's healthcare arena, complex problems warrant the development of groups. These groups may represent either individuals working in teams or multiple organizations working in a coalition. Both of these scenarios are representative of partnerships. These partnerships illustrate a working towards shared decision-making whereby participants strive to make their common vision a reality. Nurses are leaders who may initiate, coach, and mentor others as they work in groups whether these groups be team based or coalition based.

References

AIDS Coalition to Unleash Power (Act Up) (2006). *Civil disobedience training*. Retrieved from http://www.actupny.org/documents/CDdocuments/Consensus.html

Allen, J., Dyas, J., & Jones, M. (2004). Building consensus in health care: A guide to using the nominal group technique. *British Journal of Community Nursing, 9*(3), 110–114.

Bruce, R. A., & McKane, S. U. (Eds.) (2000). *Community-based public health: A partnership model*. Washington, DC: American Public Health Association.

Butterfoss, F. D. (2007). *Coalitions and partnerships in community health*. San Francisco, CA: Jossey-Bass.

Butterfoss, F. D., Goodman, R. M., & Wandersman, A. (1993). Community coalitions for prevention and health promotion. *Health Education Research, 8*(3), 315–330.

Butterfoss, F. D., & Kegler, M. C. (2009). The community coalition action theory. In R. J. DiClemente, R. A. Crosby, & M. C. Kegler (Eds.), *Emerging theories in health promotion practice and research* (pp. 237–276). San Francisco, CA: Jossey-Bass.

Cartwright, J., & Limandri, B. (1997). The challenge of multiple roles in the qualitative clinician research-participant client relationship. *Qualitative Health Research, 7*(2), 223–235.

Center for Prevention Research and Development (2006). *Evidence-based practices for effective community coalitions*. Champaign, IL: Center for Prevention Research and Development, Institute of Government and Public Affairs, University of Illinois.

Committee on Quality of Health Care in America, Institute of Medicine (2001). *Crossing the quality chasm: A new health system for the 21st century*. Washington, DC: National Academies Press.

Committee on the Robert Wood Johnson Foundation Initiative on the Future of Nursing at the Institute of Medicine (2011). *The future of nursing: Leading change, advancing health*. Washington, DC: National Academies Press.

Conflict Research Consortium (1998). *International online training program on intractable conflict: Consensus building*. Retrieved from http://www.colorado.edu/conflict/peace/treatment/consens.htm

Cramer, M. E., Atwood, J. R., & Stoner, J. A. (2006). A conceptual model for understanding effective coalitions involved in health promotion programing. *Public Health Nursing, 23*(1), 67–73.

Cronenwett, L., Sherwood, G., Barnsteiner, J., Disch. J., Johnson, J., Mitchell, P., et al. (2007). Quality and safety education for nurses. *Nursing Outlook, 55*(3), 122–131.

Feighery, E., & Rogers, T. (1990). *Building and maintaining effective coalitions*. Retrieved from http://www.ttac.org/tcn/peers/pdfs/07.24.12/CA_BuildingAndMaintainingEffectiveCoalitions_Resource.pdf

Finkelman, A., & Kenner, C. (2010). *Professional nursing concepts: Competencies for quality leadership*. Sudbury, MA: Jones & Bartlett Learning.

Foster-Fishman, P. G., Berkowitz, S. L., Lounsbury, D. W., Jacobson, S., & Allen, N. A. (2001). Building collaborative capacity in community coalitions: A review and integrative framework. *American Journal of Community Psychology, 29*(2), 241–261.

Gadamer, H. G. (1976). *Philosophical hermeneutics* (D. Linge, Trans. & Ed.). Los Angeles: University of California Press.

Greiner, A. C., & Knebel, E. (2003). *Health professions education: A bridge to quality.* Washington, DC: National Academies Press.

Greitemeyer, T., Schulz-Hardt, S., Brodbeck, F., & Frey, D. (2006). Information sampling and group decision-making: The effects of an advocacy decision procedure and task experience. *Journal of Experimental Psychology: Applied, 22*(1), 31–42.

Huber, D. (2006). *Leadership and nursing care management.* Philadelphia: Saunders Elsevier.

Institute of Medicine (IOM) (1972). *Educating for the health team.* Washington, DC: National Academy of Sciences.

Interprofessional Education Collaborative Expert Panel (IPEC) (2011). *Core competencies for interprofessional collaborative practice: Report of an expert panel.* Washington, DC: Interprofessional Education Collaborative.

Kang, R. (1997). Building community capacity for health promotion: A challenge for public health nurses. In B. W. Spradley & J. A. Allender (Eds.), *Readings in community health nursing* (pp. 221–241). New York: Lippincott.

Kaye, G., & Wolff, T. (Eds.) (2002). *From the ground up: A workbook on coalition building and community development.* Amherst, MA: Area Health Education Center (AHEC) /Community Partners.

Keller, L. O., Strohschein, S., & Briske, L. (2008). Population-based public health nursing practice: The intervention wheel. In M. Stanhope & J. Lancaster (Eds.), *Public health nursing: Population-centered health care in the community* (pp. 187–214). St. Louis, MO: Mosby Elsevier.

Kohn, L. T., Corrigan, J. M., & Donaldson, M. S. (Eds.) (2000). *To err is human: Building a safer health system.* Washington, DC: National Academies Press.

Légaré, F., Stacey, D., Briére, N., Desroches, S., Dumont, S., Fraser, K., Murray, M. A., Sales, A., & Aubé, D. (2011). A conceptual framework for interprofessional shared decision making in home care: Protocol for a feasibility study. *BMC: Health Services Research,* 11(23), p. 1–7. doi:10.1186/1472-6963-11-23.

Légaré, F., Stacey, D., Pouliot, S., Gauvin, F-P., Desroches, S., Kryworuchko, J., Dunn, S., Elwyn, G., Frosch, D., Gagnon. M-P., Harrison, M. B., Pluye, P., & Grahm, I. D. (2011). Interprofessionalism and shared decision-making in primary care: A stepwise approach towards a new model. *Journal of Interprofessional Care,* 25, 18–25.

Mansbridge, J. (2003). Consensus in context: A guide for social movements. In P. G. Coy (Ed.), *Consensus decision making, Northern Ireland and indigenous movements* (Vol. 24, pp. 229–253). St. Louis, MO: Elsevier Science Ltd.

Michaels, C. L. (2002). Circle communication: An old form of communication useful for 21st century leadership. *Nursing Administration Quarterly,* 26(5), 1–10.

Osmond, J. (n.d.). *Community coalition action theory as a framework for partnership development*. Retrieved from http://www.google.com/url?sa=t&rct=j&q=&esrc=s&source=web&cd=1&ved=0CDMQFjAA&url=http%3A%2F%2Fwww.dshs.state.tx.us%2Fwellness%2FPDF%2Fccat-10.29.08.pdf&ei=YLeCUuKOMK_gsATKooC4Cw&usg=AFQjCNFrfc5XD6f1HEYenyX3nEgFRIv0WQ&sig2=6khVMuNmwW9VHUMANgIcYg&bvm=bv.56343320,d.cWc

Porter-O'Grady, T., & Malloch, K. (2011). *Quantum leadership: Advancing innovation, transforming health care* (3rd ed.), Sudbury, MA: Jones & Bartlett Learning.

Senge, R., Kleiner, A., Roberts, C., Ross, R., Roth, G., & Smith, B. (1999). *The dance of change: The challenges to sustaining momentum in learning organizations*. New York: Doubleday.

Sullivan, E. J., & Decker, P. J. (2005). *Effective leadership and management in nursing*. Upper Saddle River, NJ: Prentice Hall.

Sullivan, T. (1998). *Collaboration: A health care imperative*. New York: McGraw-Hill.

Truglio-Londrigan, M. (2013). Shared decision-making in home-care from the nurse's perspective: sitting at the kitchen table—a qualitative descriptive study. *Journal of Clinical Nursing*. doi: 10.1111/jocn.12075.

U.S. Department of Health and Human Services, Agency for Healthcare Research and Quality (n.d.). *About TeamSTEPPS*. Retrieved from http://teamstepps.ahrq.gov/about-2cl_3.htm

Wald, A. (2013). Working together: Collaboration, coalition building, and community organizing. In M. Truglio-Londrigan & S. B. Lewenson (Eds.), *Public health nursing: Practicing population-based care* (2nd ed., pp. 297–313). Burlington, MA: Jones & Bartlett Learning.

Woehrle, L. M. (2003). Claims-making and consensus in collective group processes. In P. G. Coy (Ed.), *Consensus decision-making, Northern Ireland and indigenous movements* (Vol. 24, pp. 3–30). St. Louis, MO: Elsevier Science Ltd.

Yoder-Wise, P. S. (2003). *Leading and managing in nursing*. St. Louis, MO: Mosby.

Chapter 9

Evidence-Based Decision-Making

Jason T. Slyer, Catherine M. Concert, and Joanne K. Singleton

Decision-making is at the center of healthcare delivery. How should clinical decisions be made? Are decisions organizationally focused and driven? Are there inconsistencies in practice? Are clinical decisions paralyzed to change with the status quo as the practice standard? Are professional knowledge, practice, and research interwoven into the decision-making process? Are multidisciplinary teams communicating healthcare evidence with an interprofessional approach to decisions and quality initiatives? Reflecting on current practices and answering these questions can be a real eye opener. Using an interprofessional approach to clinical practice enhances patient outcomes when research evidence is used in a judicious manner. The challenge is to discover and appraise the evolving evidence base around the decisions to be made.

This chapter describes how research evidence supports decision-making and is critical for quality, professional health care and nursing practice. Making clinical decisions requires the application of theoretical knowledge and research to clinical situations (Rashotte & Carnevale,

2004). Typically, decisions are based on the knowledge attained during professional education combined with clinical experience, both in school and in practice. Although experience is an important component of the decision-making process, there is growing support in the health professions for combining the healthcare practitioner's knowledge and clinical experience with current research-based evidence. Clinical decisions are often made under uncertainty, but the extent of uncertainty diminishes when relevant and valid evidence is available to support those decisions (McNeil, 2001). Evidence-based practice (EBP) helps healthcare practitioners ask clinically pertinent questions, provides a framework for evaluating research, and encourages healthcare practitioners to incorporate research with clinical expertise (Straus & Sackett, 1998). EBP employs a systematic approach for analysis, synthesis, and evaluation of current research to determine its clinical relevance while being respectful of a patient's values and perspective, and then applying the research evidence to practice. Ultimately, the goal of EBP is to translate research into practice.

History and Definition of EBP

In 1972 Archie Cochrane, a British epidemiologist, criticized the medical profession for not providing critiques of research so policy makers and organizations could make sound decisions about health care. Cochrane advocated for the use of evidence from randomized controlled trials that would provide more scientifically valid information than other sources of evidence. Because of his influence, the Cochrane Collaboration was established in 1992 to develop, maintain, and update systematic clinical reviews of research (Cochrane Collaboration, 2010).

In 1992, a team of medical professionals led by Gordon Guyatt from McMaster University coined the term *evidence-based medicine* (EBM). EBM has been described as "the conscientious, explicit, and judicious use of current best evidence in making decisions about the care of individual patients. . . . [EBM integrates] clinical expertise with the best available external clinical evidence from systematic research" (Sackett, Rosenberg, Gray, Haynes, & Richardson, 1996, p. 71). EBP developed into a process that integrates "the best research evidence with our clinical expertise and our patient's unique values and circumstances" (Straus, Glasziou, Richardson, & Haynes, 2011, p. 1). The aim of this decision-making approach is to integrate research-based evidence into clinical practice to improve patient care and clinical outcomes.

The term EBM evolved to include other terms such as *evidence-based nursing* (EBN) and *evidence-based practice* (EBP) as systems developed to implement research evidence into an integrative approach in other healthcare disciplines, such as nursing (Hockenberry, Wilson, & Barrera, 2006; Melnyk & Fineout-Overholt, 2002), occupational therapy (Hockenberry et al., 2006; Tickle-Degnen, 1999), physical therapy (Maher, Sherrington, Elkins, Herbert, & Moseley, 2004), and speech-language pathology (Johnson, 2006; Yorkston et al., 2001).

Scott and McSherry (2009) comprehensively searched the literature for an EBN practice definition. From this search, an EBN definition was synthesized as "an ongoing process by which evidence, nursing theory and the practitioners' clinical expertise are critically evaluated and considered, in conjunction with patient involvement, to provide delivery of optimum nursing care for the individual" (Scott & McSherry, 2009, p. 1089). Buysse, Wesley, Snyder, and Winton (2006) defined EBP as "a decision-making process that integrates the best available evidence with family and professional wisdom and values" (p. 12), making it analogous to the definition of EBM. Similarly, Fineout-Overholt, Melnyk, and Schultz (2005) refer to EBP as a problem-solving approach to clinical care that integrates the conscientious use of evidence from "well-designed studies, the clinician's expertise and the patient's values and preferences" (p. 335). Inclusively, these definitions incorporate patient preferences and the application of the healthcare practitioner's expertise as essential to making the best clinical decisions. Evidence alone is insufficient for making clinical decisions. Clinical decisions should be based on a comparison of the benefits and risks, patient inconvenience, and costs combined with a consideration of the patient's values (Guyatt & Rennie, 2002).

The EBP Process

As the call to improve quality and patient outcomes intensifies, healthcare professionals are learning to utilize research evidence, in addition to their own expertise, while considering individual patient preferences, values, and beliefs to guide healthcare practices. The practice of EBP involves engaging in a systematic process of finding and utilizing the best evidence to support clinical practices. Straus et al. (2011) outlined a five-step process for employing EBP:

1. Ask a relevant clinically focused question.
2. Identify the best available evidence that answers the question.
3. Critically appraise the evidence for validity, effectiveness, and clinical usefulness.
4. Integrate the evidence into clinical practice incorporating patient values and beliefs.
5. Evaluate the effectiveness of the evidence in the clinical application for replication and sustainability.

Through this process healthcare practitioners can form answerable questions, and by identifying evidence they can find support to improve decision-making to achieve favorable patient outcomes. The best research evidence is methodologically sound and based on clinically relevant information that incorporates cost, safety, and the intervention's effectiveness, including the risks, the benefits, and the patient's perspectives (DiCenso, 2003). EBP offers a systematic framework and a set of tools for making decisions. Implementing the EBP process can foster individual healthcare practitioners, the interprofessional team, and the healthcare environment to collaboratively achieve and improve patient outcomes.

Asking Clinical Questions

Asking a well-designed clinically focused question is fundamental to the practice of EBP. Questions should be directly relevant to a practice problem at hand and phrased in a way that will guide in the search for relevant answers. A good clinical question focuses on how to improve the care of a particular patient. In contrast, a research question generates knowledge that is generalizable to a population and guides practice from a broader perspective (Fineout-Overholt et al., 2005).

One way to formulate a pertinent clinical question is to use the PICO mnemonic. The elements of a PICO question include: the *population* of interest (P), the *intervention* being investigated or *issue* of interest (I), the *comparator* or alternative intervention or issue (C), and the *outcome(s)* of interest (O). Occasionally the time it takes for an outcome to be achieved is important to the clinical question and the PICO mnemonic is modified to PICOT to include the *time* component (T). For questions of an experiential nature the PICo mnemonic is used to identify the *population* (P), the phenomena of *interest* (I), and the *context* (Co). A well-formulated PICO(T) or PICo question simplifies the identification and combination of appropriate terms to search the available literature for relevant answers to inform practice.

Identifying the Evidence

Finding the research evidence is time consuming for busy healthcare practitioners, managers, and policy makers. Electronic databases, systematic reviews, and journals are viable resources for searching and reviewing relevant information. Assessing the evidence can be a beneficial journey to better outcomes, interprofessional teamwork, and interprofessional sharing and relationships. Search engines of literature databases allow healthcare practitioners to search the literature to answer particular questions (White, 2004).

Through organizations such as the Cochrane Collaboration, the Johanna Briggs Institute, and the Campbell Collaboration, worldwide research that has been appraised and summarized is available online for healthcare practitioners to aid in decision-making. The Cochrane Collaboration (n.d.) database, known as the *Cochrane Library*, contains systematic reviews of randomized controlled trials and high-level research on a variety of healthcare issues. The Cochrane Collaboration (n.d.) promotes public access to systematic reviews for individuals generating interventions and making healthcare decisions by providing the most up-to-date research studies. The Joanna Briggs Institute (JBI, n.d.) is an international collaboration dedicated to improving worldwide healthcare outcomes. This multidisciplinary collaboration includes nursing, medical, and allied health researchers; healthcare practitioners; academics; and quality leaders in 40 countries across every continent. JBI is known for providing dependable high-level evidence to health professionals. The *JBI Database of Systematic Reviews and Implementation Reports* publishes systematic reviews containing quantitative, qualitative, economic, and/or text and opinion data that fulfill the criteria established by the Joanna Briggs Institute and its international collaborating centers and groups. The Campbell Collaboration, named after Donald Campbell, an American psychologist, is another international organization that formulates and circulates research evidence in the form of systematic reviews, published in the *Campbell Library*, in the fields of education, criminal justice, social policy, and social care (Davies & Boruch, 2001). The Campbell Collaboration's mission is "to provide high quality, sound evidence for policymakers, practitioners, and the public to make well informed decisions about public policy" (Davies & Boruch, 2001, p. 295).

Clinical practice guidelines are quality-improving strategies that promote best practices. They help healthcare practitioners by bringing together the evidence and knowledge for decision-making about a specific health condition. According to Sackett et al. (1996), good clinical guidelines have three properties. First, they characterize practice questions and identify the decision options and outcomes. Second, they identify, evaluate, and summarize the evidence in a format that is most relevant to decision makers. Third, they identify the decision points where evidence should be integrated with clinical experience in making decisions. Therefore, they identify a range of potential decisions and provide the evidence that, when added to individual clinical judgment and the patient's values and expectations, will help in determining and making the best decision for the patient (Straus et al., 2011).

Additionally, there are many databases that allow healthcare practitioners to search the literature for answers to their practice questions. The Cumulative Index to Nursing and Allied Health Literature

(CINAHL) database indexes more than 3,075 journals from the fields of nursing, allied health, alternative health, and community medicine (EBSCO Publishing, n.d.). The MEDLINE/PubMed database, produced by the National Library of Medicine, indexes more than 5,600 journals in the life sciences (U.S. National Library of Medicine, 2011). The PsycINFO database, produced by the American Psychological Association, indexes more than 2,500 journals from the behavioral sciences and mental health fields (American Psychological Association, n.d.). **Table 9-1** contains a selection of evidence-based resources. Getting to know a reference librarian at a library affiliated with your institution can provide healthcare practitioners with valuable assistance in navigating these vast databases and locating relevant evidence to answer the questions at hand.

Critically Appraising the Evidence

Critically appraising the evidence is an important step in the EBP process. Decisions for clinical practice should be made based on the

Table 9-1

Selected Evidence-Based Practice Resources

Agency for Healthcare Quality	www.ahrq.gov
The Campbell Collaboration	www.campbellcollaboration.org
Centre for Evidence-Based Medicine (University of Oxford)	www.cebm.net
Centre for Evidence-Based Medicine (Toronto)	ktclearinghouse.ca/cebm/
Centre for Reviews and Dissemination	www.crd.york.ac.uk/inst/crd
Clinical Evidence	www.clinicalevidence.org/x/index.html
The Cochrane Collaboration	www.cochrane.org
Essential Evidence Plus	www.essentialevidenceplus.com
Evidence-Based Nursing	http://ebn.bmj.com
First Consult	www.firstconsult.com
The Joanna Briggs Institute	www.joannabriggs.edu.au
National Guideline Clearinghouse	www.guideline.gov
PubMed	www.ncbi.nlm.nih.gov/pubmed/
TRIP Database (Turning Research into Practice)	www.tripdatabase.com
UpToDate	www.uptodate.com
Agency for Healthcare Research and Quality's Prevention and Chronic Care Program	www.ahrq.gov/professionals/prevention-chronic-care/index.html

highest quality evidence available. There are multiple forms of evidence. Depending on the nature of the question asked, the best evidence to answer the question may be of a quantitative or qualitative nature. For this chapter the authors will focus on quantitative evidence. Quantitative research designs can be arranged in a hierarchical fashion based on their ability to control for error and to support a cause-and-effect relationship. Numerous examples of hierarchies exist. Most of the hierarchies are centered on the magnitude of effect sizes (as in meta-analysis), sample size, randomization, blinding, and Type I and II error rates. **Figure 9-1** depicts study designs that make up a typical hierarchy. The highest level of evidence in the hierarchy is meta-analyses and systematic reviews that synthesize several studies to determine an overall effect. The next level includes randomized or pseudo-randomized controlled trials. Cohort and case-control trials involve following a group over time either prospectively or retrospectively. The lowest level incorporates the consideration of anecdotal findings such as case studies or expert opinion. It is important to remember that although the randomized controlled trial is seen as providing a high level of evidence, not all questions can be adequately answered with this type of research design.

Figure 9-1

Hierarchy of Evidence

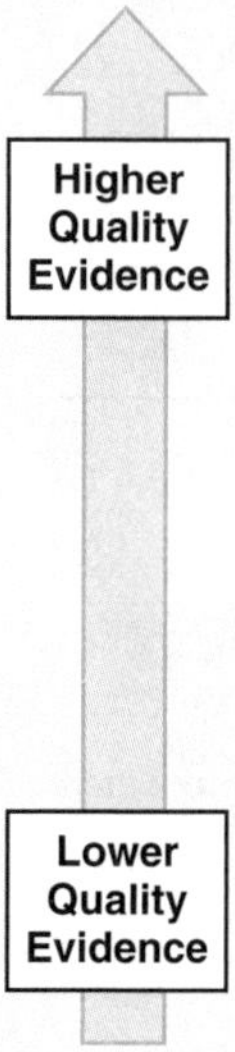

	Study design	Description
Higher Quality Evidence	Meta-analysis	A type of systematic review that combines data from different studies. It is used to determine effective treatments and plan further research.
	Systematic reviews	Systematic reviews summarize research that addresses similar research questions. Reviews employ a systematic search and a critical appraisal of the literature.
	Randomized controlled trials (RCT)	An experiment where individuals are randomly assigned into intervention or control groups.
	Cohort studies	Cohort studies utilize groups of exposed and unexposed individuals who are followed up for specific outcomes. They can be prospective or retrospective.
	Case control studies	Studies in which patients with a condition are compared to those who do not have the condition.
	Case reports	Information based on the report of one case. Often the case describes the treatment of a rare condition.
Lower Quality Evidence	Expert opinion	Information based on the opinion of experts in the field.

When critically appraising literature, there are three questions to ask about any kind of research (Melnyk & Fineout-Overholt, 2011; Oxman, Sackett, & Guyatt, 1993):

1. Are the results valid?
2. Are the results reliable?
3. Are the results applicable to the current situation?

The validity refers to whether the study results were obtained through rigorous scientific methods that minimize bias and confounding variables, permitting a high level of support for an inference. Reliability pertains to the consistency and repeatability of findings across studies (Shadish, Cook, & Campbell, 2002). Lastly, in order to transfer clinical research to patient care, the study must apply to clinical practice.

Numerous tools are available for critically appraising the validity of the available evidence (See **Table 9-2** for a selection of critical appraisal tools.) These tools contain a checklist of criteria specific to the type of study being appraised. It is important to select the appropriate tool for the research design of a study so that the appraisal criteria being used are relevant to the study being appraised. Based on whether a study meets predetermined criteria while minimizing the risk of bias, healthcare practitioners can determine if the study is of adequate quality to guide clinical decision-making.

The purpose of critical appraisal is to identify potential sources of bias. There are four main biases that may weaken a study (Joanna Briggs Institute, 2011):

Table 9-2

Critical Appraisal Instruments	
Appraisal of Guidelines Research and Evaluation (AGREE)	www.agreetrust.org
Centre for Evidence Based Medicine (University of Oxford)	www.cebm.net/index.aspx?o=1157
Critical Appraisal Skills Programme (CASP)	www.casp-uk.net
Dartmouth Biomedical Libraries	www.dartmouth.edu/~library/biomed/guides/research/ebm-teach.html?mswitch-redir=classic#critical
The Joanna Briggs Institute	www.joannabriggs.org/sumari.html www.joannabriggs.org/assets/docs/sumari/ReviewersManual-2011.pdf http://connect.jbiconnectplus.org/Appraise.aspx

- Selection bias occurs when the groups being compared are different.
- Performance bias occurs when there are differences between groups in the way an intervention is administered.
- Detection bias occurs when the outcomes are assessed differently depending on whether a participant received the intervention or the control.
- Attrition bias occurs when participants that drop out of a study are different from those remaining.

Being aware of potential sources of bias and how bias impacts the findings of a study aids healthcare practitioners in determining if the available evidence is sufficient to influence decision-making and improve practice.

Integrating the Evidence into Practice

It may take many years to translate research findings into clinical practice. Several organizations and federal agencies are placing an emphasis on accelerating the translation of research to practice (Clancy, Slutsky, & Patton, 2004). There are a number of models and frameworks to facilitate the transfer of research into clinical practice (Langley et al., 2009; Rycroft-Malone & Bucknall, 2010). Some examples include:

- The Iowa model of EBP is a practice model in which interprofessional teams critique and synthesize research findings for use in changing practices and improving outcomes. If evidence is lacking, consideration moves toward conducting a research study.
- The Advancing Research and Clinical practice through close Collaboration (ARCC) model is a conceptual framework to guide system-wide implementation and sustainability of EBP to improve outcomes through creation of an EBP culture and removal of barriers to EBP.
- The Joanna Briggs Institute model for evidence utilization is a descriptive framework for practice change that describes how to synthesize and embed evidence into practice and evaluate the outcomes of utilizing evidence within the health system.
- The PDSA (Plan, Do, Study, Act) framework is a trial-and-learn methodology in which research evidence is incorporated into a plan to improve practice, data is collected and analyzed to determine whether the practice change resulted in an improvement, and actions are formulated based on what was learned during the change cycle.

The work of the Institute of Medicine (IOM, 2001), a nonprofit organization responsible for helping healthcare professionals navigate the best evidence for high quality decision-making, is significant to the U.S. healthcare system because it provides a means for integrating information to improve practice modalities. The IOM's work encourages and challenges healthcare practitioners to rethink traditional ways of practice (Melnyk, Fineout-Overholt, Stillwell, & Williamson, 2010). Effective solutions focus on promoting quality research evidence for relevant decision-making and clinical practice. Continuous education of healthcare professionals is essential for decision-making. Identifying opportunities for change requires research evidence that supports effective and efficient decisions. Implementation of a sophisticated process will change an outdated practice by augmenting it with the best research evidence, giving healthcare practitioners a greater opportunity to move practice forward.

Although the IOM strategized the decision-making process for healthcare professionals, there continues to be room for improvement. Quality initiatives from other agencies such as The Joint Commission (TJC), Institute for Healthcare Improvement (IHI), American Nurses Credentialing Center (ANCC), and National Database of Nursing Quality Indicators (NDNQI) have been developed. Third-party payers, businesses, patients, and the government are in full support of the EBP process. These organizations and systems have encouraged healthcare practitioners and facilities to promote collaboration and communication, close gaps, and uncover new ways of looking at quality through evidence and practice. The use of information technology bolsters the search for alternative strategies, aiding healthcare professionals to access an enormous amount of methodical evidence and transform it into practice.

With the advent of nursing excellence, Magnet designation, and acceleration in education and educational competencies, a worldview of EBP has emerged. A multitude of evidence has gained strength as new research evidence is evolving. Significant research evidence guides decision-making and nursing practice. Incorporating individual patient experiences into this process will lead to measurable outcomes. EBP is collaborative. It is essential for various disciplines to establish an interprofessional approach to research evidence, thereby applying and translating the best evidence to clinical situations and decision-making. For health care to be individualized and dynamic, critical strategies and meaningful EBP must be supported despite indecisions and probable outcomes. Nurses need to be proactive, inquisitive, change agents, and on the forefront of nursing practice. Obtaining the best available evidence for quality nursing and health care is the cornerstone to enhancing the decision-making process.

Healthcare professionals need to collaborate continually to promote an interprofessional approach to relevant decisions. Decisions are judgments based on knowledge acquired during a combination of professional training and lifelong clinical experience. Clinical decisions are made when practitioners look at uncertainty through a different lens by applying theoretical knowledge with critical appraisal and translation of the evidence into clinical practice. Clinical expertise, care quality, educational coordination, and interprofessional collaboration will be essential knowledge and skills to meet the demands for EBP. Effective communication can promote safety, best practices, and improved healthcare performance. Challenging the status quo involves movement to remove interprofessional barriers while working toward identification, sharing, and recognition of best practices (Meleis, 2010). Appreciative inquiry provides a way to reframe the focus and language in a more positive way (Preskill & Catsambas, 2006). One of the key elements of appreciative inquiry is the implementation of change that focuses on the positive, what works best, what is possible, and the involvement of all individuals on the interprofessional team. The significant challenge is how to create, within the existing and future healthcare environment, the competency to work in teams capable of effective collaboration and guidance of patients through primary health care processes and complex systems. Advancing and sustaining continuity of care while using comprehensive technology and innovations can enhance the patient experience and demonstrate the best healthcare outcomes supported by evidence-based research.

Current research is vast and limitless. Searching for best practices is laborious. The best evidence is usually found in clinically relevant research that has been conducted using sound methodology (Sackett & Haynes, 2002). Healthcare practitioners today must continuously review the literature for the best evidence. Knowing the process, obtaining the evidence, and understanding study designs are significant components to identifying relevant information and decision-making. Depending on the clinical situation, healthcare practitioners can apply research evidence to a specific clinical decision or to an entire population after considering whether or not all can benefit from the intervention.

Evaluating the Effectiveness of Evidence in Practice

Decisions made based on evidence from the literature should not go directly into practice without an evaluation of their effectiveness within a current practice situation and organizational system. Significant research findings may not be generalizable to all practice situations, as differences inherently exist between settings and populations. Using one of the practice change models, such as the PDSA cycle mentioned above, healthcare professions can utilize small, rapid cycle tests of change to evaluate the effectiveness of a change based on best evidence in current practice settings. These rapid cycle tests call for an evaluation of the change process on a subset of the population over short time periods. Process and outcome measures should be collected to determine the impact of the change. The knowledge learned through these small tests of change should be evaluated and adjustments made to the practice change when suspected outcomes are not achieved. Multiple small cycle tests of change are usually needed to ensure replication and sustainability of a change prior to rolling out the change on a larger scale.

Evidence-based decision-making will continue to evolve; the process, interprofessional team growth, and interprofessional approach will change as the entire process, practice, and patient values interact with the evidence. The wisdom gained from developing innovations and new paradigms is based on knowing the value of the evidence discovered.

Barriers to Evidence-Based Practice

Barriers have been identified that may prevent the use of EBP. An EBP culture may be difficult to establish because healthcare practitioners may lack the ability to identify, obtain, and critically evaluate information. Additionally, the time pressures of clinical practice and organizational barriers may diminish the application of evidence in clinical practice.

Pravikoff, Tanner, and Pierce (2005) surveyed 760 nurses in the United States to ascertain whether nurses were aware of the need for research-based information, if they had the ability to find resources, and if the resources were available. Their findings indicated that the majority of nurses are aware of the need for information but frequently sought information from a colleague rather than from research. Nurses believe they are not adequately prepared to search for, appraise, and interpret research to aid in clinical decision-making.

Solomon and Spross (2011) conducted an integrative literature review to examine barriers to EBP. Common barriers from the 23 studies identified in this review echoed the findings of the nurses surveyed in the Pravikoff et al. (2005) study. Barriers included time constraints, specifically time to locate and read evidence; the lack of authority to change practice; difficulty accessing research; and a lack of confidence in the ability to evaluate research and interpret statistics and research language.

With the potential for EBP to improve the quality of healthcare delivery, it is important for healthcare practitioners to adopt EBP to promote best practices and avoid variations in care that can lead to errors (Stevens & Staley, 2006). Changing the organizational culture to encourage the integration of EBP requires administrative support. Support for EBP must focus on its importance not only in improving healthcare quality, but also in creating an environment of inquiry and openness to foster utilization of EBP. Strategies to overcome barriers to EBP use may include EBP committees, journal clubs, clinical coaching, or collaboration among health professional students, faculty, and clinical staff (Pravikoff, 2006). Incorporating EBP philosophy and skills into job descriptions and clinical ladders highlights the importance of adopting EBP into clinical practice (Solomon & Spross, 2011). Agencies and departments should establish and promote relationships with researchers and reference librarians to aid in training healthcare practitioners and provide resources for identifying and interpreting research evidence.

Making clinical decisions entails the application of theoretical knowledge and research to clinical situations (Rashotte & Carnevale, 2004). Healthcare practitioners are educated to enhance quality of care and improve patient outcomes by making clinically relevant decisions. This process cannot be done in a silo. The purpose of EBP is to ensure care quality for each individual patient by involving the patient in the clinical decision. Healthcare practitioners will have to consider the patient's choices to proceed or hold treatment modalities because it is the right thing for that patient at that particular time. Sackett et al. (1996) indicated that EBM involves "the more thoughtful identification and compassionate use of individual patients' predicaments, rights, and preferences in making clinical decisions about their care" (p. 71). It is about understanding the entire situation, process, and practice.

Case Study 1

This case study looks at a patient with laryngeal carcinoma. A search of the literature identifies practice guidelines from the National Comprehensive Cancer Network (2012) and from leading healthcare practitioners in the field (Moyer & Wolf, 2009). From these guidelines it is determined that the patient has two possible options for curative treatment: surgical intervention or external beam radiation therapy. The guidelines demonstrate that both options are excellent for controlling laryngeal carcinoma, especially at an early stage. One consideration in this decision is that external beam radiation can preserve the patient's voice, an important aspect for quality of life. Radiation therapy, however, requires 7 weeks of daily treatment with acute side effects such as dysphasia, odynophagia, weight loss, fatigue, and pain. On the other hand, the surgical intervention could result in paralysis of the vocal cords. Advanced carcinoma may require a total laryngectomy, leaving the patient with an opening in the throat (stoma). If a laryngectomy is performed, a feeding tube is necessary for nutritional intake. Additionally, there will be alteration in speech requiring speech and swallowing therapy to learn how to speak through the stoma. Quality of life and activities of daily living can be limited with surgical intervention.

The decision-making process necessitates discussion of these physical and psychosocial aspects with the patient. The patient will need to decide on the course of treatment; the healthcare practitioner can summarize all the options, patient outcomes, risks, and benefits from each choice, and the research evidence supporting each treatment option. The patient's individual preferences will weigh heavily on the decision. Recommendations for individual patients can also be based on anatomic, clinical, and social issues integrated into the decision-making process using an interprofessional shared decision-making approach.

Case Study 2

A nurse practitioner working in a heart failure disease management clinic manages a caseload of adult patients with varying degrees of heart failure. The majority of this practitioner's patients have a left ventricular ejection fraction of less than 40% and are classified as New York Heart Association function class III (comfortable at rest but symptoms with less than ordinary activity). This patient population is prone to frequent bouts of symptom exacerbation leading to rehospitalizations. The nurse practitioner is aware that her hospital is now losing Medicare reimbursement because of its high heart failure readmission rates. The nurse practitioner needs to evaluate their current practice to see if changes can be made to reduce the readmission rate for her patients.

The nurse practitioner currently utilizes heart failure practice guidelines developed by the Heart Failure Society of America (Lindenfeld et al., 2010). These guidelines are based on a synthesized review of the literature; recommendations for practice are made by an expert panel that reviews the research and updates the recommendations. These guidelines address topics related to the prevention, evaluation, and management of patients with heart failure. The recommendations are weighted according to the source of the evidence, with randomized controlled trials being considered the highest strength and expert opinion the lowest strength. The guideline authors considered all levels of evidence in making the best recommendations for practice.

Although the guidelines make specific recommendations for discharge criteria and planning for hospital discharge, there are no specific recommendations other than "follow-up by phone or clinic visit early after discharge" (Lindenfeld et al., 2010, p. 500) to try to reduce readmission after a patient has been discharged. The nurse practitioner then decides to search the literature for an answer to the question of how best to reduce readmission rates for their patients.

The search of the literature identifies a systematic review on the effectiveness of nurse-coordinated transitioning of care on readmission rates for patients with heart failure (Slyer, Concert, Eudebio, Rogers, & Singleton, 2011). This systematic review identified 16 randomized controlled trials that evaluated transitioning of care processes. Ten studies showed a reduction in readmission rates, especially when interventions utilized home visits or home visits coupled with telephone follow-up.

The nurse practitioner took this evidence and developed a plan to team up with a local home care agency to follow up on patients after discharge. A plan for in-home follow-up for eligible patients by the home care agency and telephone follow-up by the nurse practitioner was devised. The plan was put into action and readmission rates would be reassessed after 1 month. The nurse practitioner and the home care agency would analyze their results after this 1-month test of change, make any adjustments to the plan as needed, and retest the changes in another month-long cycle.

Conclusion

Clinical decisions about patient care should be based on the best research evidence available. The best research evidence refers to methodologically sound and clinically relevant research that incorporates the cost, safety, and effectiveness of interventions with risks and benefits, as well as patient perspectives (DiCenso, 2003). EBP offers a systematic framework and a set of tools for making clinical decisions. By implementing the process of EBP, individual healthcare practitioners, as well as institutions, foster an EBP environment that has the potential to improve patient care. Interprofessional teams, utilizing an EBP framework, will shape the future of accountable health care through improved quality, safety, and outcomes.

References

American Psychological Association (n.d.). *PsycINFO*. Retrieved from http://www.apa.org/pubs/databases/psycinfo/index.aspx

Buysse, V., Wesley, P. W., Snyder, P., & Winton, P. (2006). Evidence-based practice: What does it really mean for the early childhood field? *Young Exceptional Children, 9*(4), 2–11.

Clancy, C. M., Slutsky, J. R., & Patton, L. T. (2004). Evidence-based health care 2004: AHRG moves research to translation and implementation. *Health Services Research, 39*(5), xv–xxiv.

Cochrane Collaboration (n.d.). *The Cochrane database of systematic reviews*. Retrieved from http://www.cochrane.org

Cochrane Collaboration (2010). *Archie Cochrane: The name behind the Cochrane Collaboration*. Retrieved from http://www.cochrane.org/about-us/history/archie-cochrane

Davies, P., & Boruch, R. (2001). The Campbell Collaboration does for public policy what Cochrane does for health. *British Medical Journal, 323*(7308), 294–295.

DiCenso, A. (2003). Evidence-based nursing practice: How to get there from here. *Nursing Leadership, 16*(4), 20–26.

EBSCO Publishing (n.d.). *The CINAHL database*. Retrieved from http://www.ebscohost.com/biomedical-libraries/the-cinahl-database

Fineout-Overholt, E., Melnyk, B. M., & Schultz, A. (2005). Transforming health care from the inside out: Advancing evidence-based practice in the 21st century. *Journal of Professional Nursing, 21*(6), 335–344.

Guyatt, G., & Rennie, D. (2002). *Users' guide to the medical literature: Essentials of evidence-based practice*. Chicago: American Medical Association (AMA) Press.

Hockenberry, M., Wilson, D., & Barrera, P. (2006). Implementing evidence-based nursing practice in a pediatric hospital. *Pediatric Nursing, 32*(4), 371–377.

Institute of Medicine (IOM) (2001). *Crossing the quality chasm: A new health system for the 21st century*. Washington, DC: National Academies Press.

Johanna Briggs Institute (JBI) (n.d.). *JBI database of systematic reviews and implementation reports*. Retrieved from http://www.joannabriggslibrary.org/index.php/jbisrir

Joanna Briggs Institute (2011). *Joanna Briggs Institute reviewers' manual: 2011 edition*. Adelaide, South Australia: Joanna Briggs Institute.

Johnson, C. J. (2006). Getting started in evidence-based practice for childhood speech-language disorders. *American Journal of Speech-Language Pathology, 15*(1), 20–35.

Langley, G. J., Moen, R. D., Nolan, K. M., Nolan, T. W., Norman, C. L., & Provost, L. P. (2009). *The improvement guide: A practical approach to enhancing organizational performance* (2nd ed.). San Francisco, CA: Jossey-Bass.

Lindenfeld, J., Albert, N. M., Boehmer, J. P., Collins, S. P., Ezekowitz, J. A., Givertz, M. M., et al. (2010). HFSA 2010 comprehensive heart failure practice guideline. *Journal of Cardiac Failure, 16*(6), 475–539.

Maher, C. G., Sherrington, C., Elkins, M., Herbert, R. D., & Moseley, A. M. (2004). Challenges for evidence-based physical therapy: Accessing and interpreting high-quality evidence on therapy. *Physical Therapy, 84*(7), 644–654.

McNeil, B. J. (2001). Hidden barriers to improvements in the quality of care. *New England Journal of Medicine, 345*(22), 1612–1620.

Meleis, A. I. (2010). Theoretical development of transitions. In A. Meleis (Ed.), *Transitions theory: Middle-range and situation-specific theories in nursing research and practice*. New York: Springhouse.

Melnyk, B. M., & Fineout-Overholt, E. (2002). Key steps in implementing evidence-based practice: Asking compelling, searchable questions and searching for the best evidence. *Pediatric Nursing, 28*(3), 262–263, 266.

Melnyk, B. M., & Fineout-Overholt, E. (2011). *Evidence-based practice in nursing and healthcare. A guide to best practice* (2nd ed.). Philadelphia, PA: Wolters Kluwer Health/Lippincott Williams & Wilkins.

Melnyk, B. M., Fineout-Overholt, E., Stillwell, S. B., & Williamson, K. M. (2010). Evidence-based practice: Step by step: The seven steps of evidence-based practice. *American Journal of Nursing, 110*(1), 51–52.

Moyer, J. S., & Wolf, G. T. (2009). Advanced stage cancer of the larynx. Part A: General principles and management. In L. B. Harrison, R. B. Sessions, & W. K. Hong (Eds.), *Head and neck cancer: A multidisciplinary approach* (pp. 367–384). Philadelphia, PA: Lippincott Williams and Wilkins.

National Comprehensive Cancer Network (2012). *NCCN clinical practice guidelines in oncology: Cancer [v. 1.2012]*. Retrieved from http://www.nccn.org/professionals/physician_gls/pdf/head-and-neck.pdf

Oxman, A. D., Sackett, D. L., & Guyatt, G. H. (1993). Users' guides to the medical literature I. How to get started. The Evidence-Based Medicine Working Group. *Journal of the American Medical Association, 270*(17), 2093–2095.

Pravikoff, D. S. (2006). Mission critical: A culture of evidence-based practice and information literacy. *Nursing Outlook, 54*(4), 254–255.

Pravikoff, D. S., Tanner, A. B., & Pierce, S. T. (2005). Readiness of U.S. nurses for evidence-based practice. *American Journal of Nursing, 105*(9), 40–51.

Preskill, H., & Catsambas, T. (2006). *Reframing evaluation through appreciative inquiry*. Thousand Oaks, CA: Sage Publications.

Rashotte, J., & Carnevale, F. A. (2004). Medical and nursing clinical decision-making: A comparative epistemological analysis. *Nursing Philosophy, 5*(2), 160–174.

Rycroft-Malone, J., & Bucknall, T. (2010). *Models and frameworks for implementing evidence-based practice: Linking evidence to action*. West Sussex, United Kingdom: Wiley-Blackwell.

Sackett, D. L., & Haynes, R. B. (2002). The architecture of diagnosis research. *British Medical Journal, 324*(7336), 539–541.

Sackett, D. L., Rosenberg, W. M., Gray, J. A., Haynes, R. B., & Richardson, W. S. (1996). Evidence-based medicine: What it is and what it isn't. *British Medical Journal, 312*(7023), 71–72.

Scott, K., & McSherry, R. (2009). Evidence based nursing: Clarifying the concepts for nurses in practice. *Journal of Clinical Nursing, 18*(8), 1085–1095.

Shadish, W. R., Cook, T. D., & Campbell, D. T. (2002). *Experimental and quasi-experimental designs for generalized causal inference.* New York: Houghton Mifflin.

Slyer, J. T., Concert, C. M., Eudebio, A. M., Rogers, M. E., & Singleton, J. (2011). A systematic review of the effectiveness of nurse coordinated transitioning of care on readmission rates for patients with heart failure. *Joanna Briggs Institute Library of Systematic Reviews, 9*(15), 464–490.

Solomon, N. M., & Spross, J. A. (2011). Evidence-based practice barriers and facilitators from a continuous quality improvement perspective: An integrative review. *Journal of Nursing Management, 19*(1), 109–120.

Stevens, K. R., & Staley, J. M. (2006). The quality chasm reports, evidence-based practice, and nursing's response to improve healthcare. *Nursing Outlook, 54*(2), 94–101.

Straus, S. E., Glasziou, P., Richardson, W. S., & Haynes, R. B. (2011). *Evidence based medicine: How to practice and teach it* (4th ed.). London: Churchill Livingstone Elsevier.

Straus, S. E., & Sackett, D. L. (1998). Using research findings in clinical practice. *British Medical Journal, 317*(7154), 339–342.

Tickle-Degnen, L. (1999). Organizing, evaluating, and using evidence in occupational therapy practice. *American Journal of Occupational Therapy, 53*(5), 537–539.

U.S. National Library of Medicine (2011). *MEDLINE fact sheet*. Retrieved from http://www.nlm.nih.gov/pubs/factsheets/medline.html

White, B. (2004). Making evidence-based medicine doable in everyday practice. *Family Practice Management, 11*(2), 51–58.

Yorkston, K. M., Spencer, K. A., Duffy, J. R., Beukelman, D. R., Golper, L. A., Miller, R. M., et al. (2001). Evidence-based medicine and practice guidelines: Application to the field of speech-language pathology—Academy of Neurologic Communication Disorders and Sciences: Writing committee for practice guidelines in dysarthria. *Journal of Medical Speech-Language Pathology, 9*(4), 243–256.

Chapter 10

Healthcare Costs Matter: Economics and Decision-Making

Donna M. Nickitas and
Linda Berger Spivack

This chapter explains how the many decisions involving health care are driven by the realities of the economy, whether those realities are local, regional, state, or national. Nurses need to understand and interpret the concepts and issues behind healthcare finance and economic decision-making. It is these economic decisions, as well as health policy, that determine the distribution of resources for how care is rendered to individuals, families, and populations. For example, chronic conditions such as diabetes, arthritis, hypertension, and kidney disease account for 7 of 10 deaths among Americans each year and for 75 percent of the nation's health spending (Conway, Goodrich, Macklin, Sasse, & Cohen, 2011). The obesity epidemic and growing levels of preventable diseases and chronic conditions contribute greatly to the high costs of health care. Additionally, an aging population has placed increasing demands on the U.S. healthcare system to address the cost of care at the end of life in a cost-effective manner (Rice & Betcher, 2010). By understanding the economic realities of health care, nurses are better able to recognize the relationships between cost-effective preventive services and improved quality of life.

The Patient Protection and Affordable Care Act (ACA), the health insurance reform legislation passed by Congress and signed into law by President Obama on March 23, 2010, helps make prevention affordable and accessible for all Americans by requiring health insurance plans to cover recommended preventive services. Nurses have a vital role in creating opportunities for better health, better health care, and lower costs through improvement. It is crucial that they confront the cold hard facts about the growth of health spending and how it is fueling the federal budget deficit, crowding out other priorities such as education and infrastructure repairs in state budgets, restraining job growth, and jeopardizing the finances of U.S. families (Nickitas, 2013). In fact, Emanuel (2012) reports that in 2010, 29 states spent more on Medicaid than on primary and secondary education, and by the middle of 2011 another 18 states had cut funding for kindergarten through 12th grade. Healthcare costs matter!

Healthcare Spending

According to the Centers for Medicare and Medicaid Services (CMS), healthcare spending in the United States will reach nearly $5 trillion, or 20 percent of gross domestic product (GDP), by 2021 (Ginsburg et al., 2012). CMS, previously known as the Health Care Financing Administration (HCFA), is a federal agency within the U.S. Department of Health and Human Services (DHHS) that administers the Medicare program and works in partnership with state governments to administer Medicaid, the Children's Health Insurance Program (CHIP), and health insurance portability standards.

It is imperative that nurses understand and appreciate how healthcare delivery decisions are financed and determined by economic factors. The business of caring is immensely complicated, and much of it is determined by costs. If the rate of growth in healthcare expenditures is not slowed then the government will either have to raise taxes, cut other government spending, or continue to run huge deficits (Silver, 2013). "For every 10 percent increase in the average cost of family health insurance premiums, the ranks of the uninsured increased by 0.55 percent. When premiums doubled between 2000 and 2009, the percentage of Americans who were covered by employer-sponsored health insurance dropped to 61 percent from 69 percent" (Emanuel, 2012, p. A4). Money matters as it relates to healthcare access, costs, and coverage; however, costs and coverage are only half of the healthcare message. Nurses and nurse leaders still have a responsibility to advocate for health care as a basic human right and ensure access to essential health services for all (Nickitas, 2011a).

The challenge is how best to engage, empower, and entrust every nurse to become a "nurse economist" (Nickitas, 2011b). Nurses must come to appreciate the important role the economy plays in the healthcare decision-making process. In particular, nurses need to know how to use this economically driven information as they make decisions and provide care within the environmental context in which they practice. All nurses, regardless of their position, must understand, from a broad perspective, how the economy of health care as a whole is derived and driven. This chapter explores issues related to healthcare spending including nurses' understanding of healthcare finances and budgeting and cost–benefit analysis. It also explores the kind of leadership acumen that is required to make nursing and healthcare economic decisions. A case study that illustrates the application and analysis of an economic decision-making model in a healthcare setting and the subsequent effect on healthcare outcomes will be used.

Rising Healthcare Costs

Peter Orszag, former director of the Office of Management and Budget, has written that rising healthcare costs are at the core of the U.S. long-term fiscal imbalance (2011). He further suggests that no challenge in health care is more important than reducing healthcare spending.

> In 2011, US health care spending grew 3.9 percent to reach \$2.7 trillion, marking the third consecutive year of relatively slow growth. Growth in national health spending closely tracked growth in nominal gross domestic product (GDP) in 2010 and 2011, and health spending as a share of GDP remained stable from 2009 through 2011, at 17.9 percent. (Hartman, Martin, Benson, & Catlin, 2013, p. 87)

Even as growth in spending at the national level has remained stable, total personal healthcare spending growth accelerated in 2011 (from 3.7 percent to 4.1 percent), in part because of faster growth for individual spending on prescription drugs and physician and clinical services. Total U.S. healthcare spending reached \$2.7 trillion in 2011, or \$8,680 per person, representing an increase of 3.9 percent from 2010 (Hartman et al., 2013). These rising healthcare costs rivet our attention as one of the leading economic influences faced by the nursing profession.

Nurses as Drivers of Clinical and Financial Innovation

As the largest segment of the healthcare workforce, nurses need to be full partners with other health professions to achieve significant improvements at the local, state, and national levels in care delivery. As a health professional partner, nurses understand and have demonstrated expertise and experience with innovative models of care, as well as the financial, technical, and political savvy to close clinical and financial holes within a healthcare delivery system. Nurses are in a unique position to lead practice innovations that are needed to succeed clinically and financially under the ACA (Institute of Medicine [IOM], 2010). They play an essential role in supporting and realizing the vision for health care in the United States.

The ACA provides new standards for private health insurance, including identifying minimum benefits for health insurance, placing limits on cost sharing for covered benefits, and establishing new rules for private health insurance that assures coverage for individuals with health problems as well as limits premiums and contribution differences based on health-related factors (U.S. Department of Health and Human Services, 2013). Together these new provisions will seek to reduce the financial burden for those with a low income or who have significant health problems.

As hospitals and other care delivery systems move to implement changes called for in the ACA and by CMS, the focus will be on curbing costs while providing safe, quality patient-centered care. In order for professional nurses to take this lead in healthcare finance decisions and healthcare reform initiatives, however, they must be knowledgeable about the issues of costs, quality, and evidence-based care. This will require nurses to have the financial acumen to coordinate and manage persons with complex biopsychosocial healthcare needs and serve a diverse outpatient populations that will include the uninsured, those on Medicaid, and those who are geographically and/or economically disadvantaged. Additionally, nurses will need financial knowledge and information as they make the "business case" for improving and maintaining high-quality nursing care. It is up to the profession itself to develop and provide directions for public and private reimbursement systems to specifically account for the intensity of nursing care and to develop directions for nurses in a pay-for-performance environment.

Consumers Demand Quality at Reduced Costs

To effectively manage the complex needs of Americans from an access, cost, and quality perspective, the U.S. healthcare system must become more responsive. In fact, IBM's Paul Grundy recently noted that "Large corporations are now the buyers of care principally for the 65 and younger population" (Weinstock, 2012, p. 30). Major employers are increasingly factoring healthcare quality and costs into their strategic business decisions. A 2012 health benefits survey conducted by the National Business Group found that leading companies are now providing employees with more and more information about healthcare service pricing and quality. And these same companies plan to improve provider quality by offering specialty treatment or narrow networks, and providing incentives for the use of evidence-based care (Weinstock, 2012).

With U.S. healthcare costs rising not only for employers, but also for consumers and the government, the move towards a value-based business model ensuring high-quality care at the lowest price is a national goal. Adopting new payment models that embrace value-based purchasing, accountable care, and patient medical home models will help ensure high quality that strategically manages healthcare costs. This transformation process linking patient safety and quality of care to costs has been recently funded by the Centers for Medicare and Medicaid Innovation as a part of the national Partnership for Patients initiative called the Hospital Engagement Networks (HEN) project (Taylor, 2012).

One example of a HEN project is to reduce 10 targeted hospital-acquired conditions (see **Table 10-1**) by 40 percent and cut hospital readmissions by 20 percent, saving an estimated 60,000 lives over 3 years and saving $50 billion in Medicare funding over 10 years (Taylor, 2012, p. 38). Currently, more than 3,900 hospitals in 46 states have decided to participate in the 26 Hospital Engagement Networks, which were awarded $218.8 million in contracts (Taylor, 2012). These networks are required to identify measures for each hospital-acquired condition, and file monthly, quarterly, and annual reports describing their hospital's progress. The aim of this HEN project is to improve patient safety by reducing adverse events and cutting healthcare costs by 10 percent.

Changes in federal as well as state financing of the delivery system are requiring nurses to develop much broader financial acumen. This includes responding to the demands made by CMS and private healthcare insurers to provide defect-free health care as much as possible.

The challenge for nursing is to ensure that evidence-based processes and measures are translated and implemented into daily care. Nurses need to be full partners in designing and improving care, including understanding the multiple forces that drive the escalation of the healthcare expenses (IOM, 2010). Every nurse must understand that preventing errors is an investment toward quality patient care that can be fully realized and rewarded. For example, nurses must come

Table 10-1

Targeted HEN Hospital-Acquired Conditions
1. Central-line–associated bloodstream infections
2. Adverse drug events
3. Pressure ulcers
4. Injuries from falls or immobility
5. Catheter-associated urinary infections
6. Ventilator-associated pneumonia
7. Surgical-site infections
8. Venous thromboembolism
9. Obstetrical adverse events
10. Preventable readmissions

to appreciate how the cost of quality nursing care generates potential savings through the avoidance of "never" events and medication errors. This culture of economic accountability is built upon an understanding that every patient encounter is a return on investment in quality.

Not all healthcare expenses are equal; nor are the patients who incur those expenses. Americans must acknowledge how complex, uncoordinated cases drive up costs. In fact, only a small percentage of patients (1 percent), known as high-frequency users, accounted for roughly one fifth of all healthcare spending in 2009, or more than $90,000 per person according to a recently released report by the Agency for Healthcare Research and Quality (Bush, 2012, p. 31). This report revealed that 5 percent of patients accounted for half of overall healthcare costs; in contrast, 50 percent of patients accounted for only 3 percent of healthcare spending. Why is it that such a small segment of the U.S. population consumes 20 percent of society's wealth at such a massive rate? The answer is simple—health care is neither coordinated nor well understood by these high-frequency patients.

Healthcare Financing

In order to slow the rise in healthcare costs, steps must be taken to address significant problems that exist with payment, benefits, regulations, and organizations in the current healthcare system. Although our healthcare system is among the most market oriented (competitively driven) in the world, it remains the most heavily regulated sector of the U.S. economy (Conover, 2004). The regulators of the healthcare delivery system include:

- CMS utilization reviews of appropriateness
- Office of Safety and Health Administration (OSHA) inspection of workplace safety
- National Labor Relations Board monitoring of nurse unions
- National Council of State Boards of Nursing licensing exam requirements
- Limitations on medical resident or registered nurse (RN) working hours
- Fraud and abuse protections
- Managed care

Yet, despite this regulatory oversight, the United States spends almost 20 percent of its gross domestic spending on health care, compared with about half that in most developed countries (Brill, 2013). Even with this high level of spending, the results are no better than the next biggest spenders combined: Japan, Germany, France, China, the United Kingdom, Italy, Canada, Brazil, Spain, and Australia (Brill, 2013).

The Graham Center's (2005) research trend analysis projects that annual health insurance premiums will exceed the average yearly household's income in 2025 if the present rate of escalation continues. There have been many cost-containment efforts in the past but they have generally failed to reap their promised rewards. Attempts to restrain healthcare cost expansion began in 1973 with the enactment of the Health Maintenance Act (HMA). The Nixon administration instituted a "voluntary" freeze on healthcare spending initiated by the need to curtail healthcare spending during a period of double-digit inflation. Fee-for-service represented the primary method of payment between 1965 and 1983. By contrast, between the years of 1983 and 1998, a payment system based on diagnosis-related groups (DRGs), and then prospective payment systems (PPS) and later resource-based relative value (RBRV) scales dominated healthcare reimbursement. Healthcare providers reeled under the stress of declining payments, hospital bankruptcies, massive deficits, layoffs, and merger dissolutions (DeBakey, 2006; Samuel, Raleigh, Hower, & Schwartz, 2003). Government efforts to constrain advancing consumption of national economic resources moved the healthcare reimbursement system from the open-ended fee-for-service through the confines of DRGs to fully implemented managed care.

Healthcare spending grows faster than national income because the healthcare system continues to innovate and provide new treatments to individuals with serious acute and chronic illnesses. Healthcare spending is influenced by a variety of issues, including federal and state programs with differing payment systems, incentives, and reimbursement levels; private health insurers; and direct family payments for services that are covered or not covered by public and private insurance.

Over the last four decades, the average growth in healthcare spending has exceeded the growth of the economy as a whole by between 1.1 and 3.0 percentage points (Congressional Budget Office, 2013). Since 1970, healthcare spending per capita has grown at an average rate of 8.2 percent, or 2.4 percentage points faster than the gross national product (GDP). A smaller difference is projected over the 2011 to 2020 period, when the average annual growth in per capita healthcare spending (5.3 percent) is projected to be about 1.2 percentage points higher than the growth in GDP (1.4 percent) (Center for Medicare and Medicaid Services, 2010).

McKinsey researchers (as cited in Brill, 2013) reported that in 2013 healthcare spending would reach $2.8 trillion; of this total, about $800 billion will be paid by the federal government through Medicare insurance for the disabled and those 65 or older and the Medicaid program for the poor (cited in Brill, 2013). Understanding healthcare economics and healthcare public policy as it applies to the delivery of patient care is essential, including how healthcare services are reimbursed. Most healthcare services are reimbursed through Medicare, Medicaid, managed care, and third-party providers.

Health Finance

U.S. citizens enjoy a healthcare system that is fundamentally job based, with nearly two thirds of the nonelderly population receiving insurance as a job benefit (Lamb, 2004). Most healthcare costs are indirectly paid for by the consumer for care provided by hospitals and physicians. Spending on hospital care and physician services combined was $1.3 trillion in 2012 and made up just over half of healthcare expenditures (51 percent). Spending on drugs ($259.1 billion) accounts for only 10 percent of total health expenditures (The Henry J. Kaiser Family Foundation, n.d.).

The majority of U.S. healthcare consumers participate in insurance or public healthcare coverage plans. The Medicare current beneficiary survey for 1992–2002 revealed private insurance or governmental programs indirectly paid 79 percent of all healthcare costs. Only 21 percent of healthcare-related expenses were covered by individual out-of-pocket expenditure (Centers for Disease Control and Prevention [CDC], 2003). Health care is financed by income employees forego to support their employer's tax-advantaged contribution to their health insurance or the amount of state and federal taxes (roughly 20 percent) they pay to support government-funded health programs, such as Medicaid, Medicare, the Children's Health Insurance Program, the Veterans Health Administration, and federal and state public health activities.

Employees and households pay for health insurance through lower wages and higher prices. Premium growth has outpaced the growth in workers' earnings almost every year. Whereas premium increases have been between 3 and 13 percent per year since 2000, inflation and changes in workers' earnings are typically in the 2 to 4.5 percent range. This means that workers have to spend more of their income each year on health care to maintain coverage. Healthcare spending may be either direct, through increased worker contributions for premiums or related to health benefits, or indirect when employers reduce wages or limit wage increases to offset increases in premiums. There are other factors that contribute to why healthcare costs are growing faster than the economy overall, including an aging U.S. population, an increase in disease prevalence, rising levels of obesity, developments in medicine and medical technology, and expanding insurance coverage (see **Table 10-2**).

Americans must consider that the overall population growth is contributing to the increase in expenditure for health care, in particular the increase in the cohort representing individuals 65 years of age

Table 10-2

Leading Factors Driving Current Levels of Spending on Health Care
• Fee-for-service reimbursement
• Fragmentation in care delivery
• Administrative burden on providers, payers, and patients
• Population aging, rising rates of chronic disease, and comorbidities, as well as lifestyle factors and personal health choices
• Advances in medical technology
• Tax treatment of health insurance
• Insurance benefit design
• Lack of transparency about cost and quality, compounded by limited data, to inform consumer choice
• Cultural biases that influence care utilization
• Changing trends in healthcare market consolidation and competition for providers and insurers
• High unit prices of medical services
• The healthcare legal and regulatory environment, including current medical malpractice and fraud and abuse laws
• Structure and supply of the health professional workforce, including scope of practice restrictions, trends in clinical specialization, and patient access to providers

Source: http://www.rwjf.org/content/dam/farm/reports/issue_briefs/2012/rwjf401339 l, pp. 6–7. Reprinted by permission of the Bipartisan Policy Center and Paul Ginsburg.

or older, which is demonstrating the most rapid growth. Due to the advancing age of the largest cohort, the baby boomers, study projections published by the Center for Health Workforce Studies, School of Public Health at University of Albany in New York, suggest that between 2000 and 2020, the U.S. population will add 19 million older adults (Moore et al., 2005), thus adding a further strain on the healthcare system. With this growth, there is an expectation that there will be a higher volume of need for healthcare services. At the same time, while these same Americans are getting older, they are also getting sicker and more obese than in decades past. Older people have more health problems and use more health care than younger people (America's Health Insurance Plans, 2013). They expect the newest and best treatments and stand accused of overusing the healthcare system (Henderson, Meyers, Ibrahim, & Tierney, 2005).

The explosive growth in national healthcare costs is attributable to other trends as well, including an increase in disease prevalence, particularly chronic diseases such as diabetes, asthma, and heart disease, coupled with the growing ability of the health system to treat the chronically ill. For example, the rising obesity levels are driving higher levels of health spending due to other comorbidities such as heart disease or depression.

Obesity is defined by the Centers for Disease Control and Prevention (CDC) as a person having a very high amount of body fat in relation to lean body mass, or a body mass index (BMI) of 30 or greater. BMI is a measure of an adult's weight in relation to his or her height, specifically the adult's weight in kilograms divided by the square of his or her height in meters (CDC, 2006). Obesity trend data collected since 1990 reflects a gradual and unrelenting incline. In 1990, 11.6 percent of the U.S. population qualified as obese based on BMI. By 1991, only four states reported obesity prevalence rates of 15–19 percent and no states had rates at or above 20 percent. In 1995, obesity prevalence in each of the 50 states was less than 20 percent. By 2005, only four states reported obesity prevalence rates less than 20 percent, and 17 states had prevalence rates equal to or greater than 25 percent, with three of those having prevalence equal to or greater than 30 percent (CDC, 2006).

The rising incidence of obesity in the United States parallels the increasing frequency of type 2 diabetes (CDC, 2006). Individuals living with diabetes also demonstrate higher occurrences of coronary artery disease, peripheral vascular disease, major end organ damage such as renal failure, and blindness (Hogan, Dall, & Nikolov, 2003). The constellation of related medical problems associated with diabetes is associated with the increased cost of health care. Therefore, obesity and diabetes represent a rising economic impact for the individual and the healthcare system. Changes such as these, along with advancements in medical technology, diagnostic equipment, pharmaceuticals, and surgical procedures, contribute to the unrelenting rising healthcare costs (DeBakey, 2006). DeBakey (2006) further asserts that in 15 years, a projected 25 percent of federal income taxes will be used for Medicare. Government subsidies for health coverage affect cost levels and potentially cost growth. Tax subsidies for health insurance and public coverage for certain groups (poor, disabled, and elderly) reduce the costs of health care to individuals.

Patient Protection and Affordable Care Act (ACA)

The provisions provided in the ACA will affect healthcare costs by changing the way health care is covered and provided for in all types of settings, public and private. This law now includes provisions that ensure that health plans offer a core package of services known as "essential benefits." These essential benefits provide for ambulatory patient care services; emergency care; hospitalization; maternity and newborn care; pediatric services; mental health care and substance use disorder services, including behavioral health care; preventive care; rehabilitative and rehabilitative services; laboratory services; preventive and wellness services, including dental and vision care; and chronic care management.

A key feature of the ACA is that it creates new sources of healthcare coverage through state health insurances exchanges, provides for premium and cost-sharing subsidies for those with low income, expands Medicaid eligibility, makes changes to slow the growth of Medicare spending, restructures the private health insurance market, and includes numerous other health-related provisions. Exchanges are designed to allow individuals and small businesses to compare private insurance plans based on quality and price. Every state must offer an exchange but will have options on what is offered. For example, states can elect to build a fully state-based exchange, join with other states and create a regional exchange, enter into a state–federal partnership exchange, or let the federal Department of Health and Human Services (DHHS) be responsible for operating the health insurance exchange.

The health insurance exchange will combine the benefits of choice for individuals with the bargaining power and full-scale influence that's usually reserved for only large employers. These exchanges offer strong competition with the promise of lower prices and higher quality. Unlike employer-based insurance, a state health insurance exchange will offer an array of competing providers offering different plans with varying benefit levels and prices. Nurses will need to become familiar with how exchanges work, including the facts on benefits, access, and quality. Nurses can no longer ignore learning the facts about the ACA, including the new developments emerging about state health insurance exchanges. Patients will look for nurses to provide information about access to care and coverage through the exchange as well as the bare facts on how to apply, enroll, and obtain benefits. Learning about healthcare coverage is a critical skill as more and more Americans gain access to care. Nurses on the front lines of care delivery must know the basic facts about healthcare finance, including how budgets are developed and managed.

Bare Facts about Healthcare Finance and Budgets

A budget is simply a financial plan for the future. Budgets are made for both spending and revenue. Budget knowledge and responsibility help nurses become effective patient care advocates, ensuring that the patients receive the best and safest care services possible. Nurses must possess the skills and vocabulary necessary to determine what financial information is available, acquire the information needed, and interpret its impact on patient care. They must also learn what data systems are available and how best to utilize them. For many nurses, learning the language of finance and completing a budget may be riddled with fear and anxiety. At first, the terms and concepts may appear peculiar, but after the basic concepts are mastered the budgetary process becomes just as familiar as the nursing process. See **Table 10-3** for some frequently used budget terms.

To begin, each nurse must know and be able to recognize the classification of their own healthcare organizations. For example, nurses must know the difference between a for-profit healthcare organization with stockholders' equity and a not-for-profit organization with unrestricted funds or temporarily or permanently restricted funds. These classifications determine how financial outcomes are assessed, which are determined by the financial statements. A for-profit organization looks to create profitability for its stakeholders. Profitability, as a construct, is measured by the operating profit margin, or the excess of revenues over expenses (Dunham-Taylor & Pinczuk, 2010). Financial statements are required every year, and publicly traded organizations must also issue quarterly financial statements, which consist of a balance sheet, an income statement, and a cash flows statement.

Table 10-3

Frequently Used Budget Terms

- *Break-even:* the point at which the costs of operations exactly equal the revenues
- *Budget variance:* the difference between the projected budget and the actual performance
- *Full-time equivalent (FTE):* a unit of measurement that represents one person who works a full-time position—40 hours/week or 2,080 hours/year
- *Unit of service:* a measurement of specific services a patient uses within a specific time frame (e.g., patient encounters, births, operations, number of inpatients present at midnight)
- *Nursing workload:* nursing hours per patient day (NHPPD); a measurement of nursing staff labor hours needed to provide care to a patient on an inpatient unit in 24 hours
- *Relative value unit (RVU):* the complexity of a procedure
- *Overhead:* indirect costs that include such things as benefits, depreciation, administration, housekeeping, and the like
- *Product lines:* total services for a particular group of patients or similar patient diagnoses (e.g., oncology, women's health)
- *Variance analysis:* a process that enables a nurse leader to compare actual performance of a given area to the budget
- *Variance report:* a summary of the major exceptions to the budget that are experienced during a given time frame and an explanation of why the exceptions happened

Accounting Principles

The accounting principles used by for-profit organizations consist of the following formula:

$$\text{assets} = \text{liabilities} + \text{equity}$$

For not-for-profit organizations it is

$$\text{assets} = \text{liabilities} + \text{net assets or fund balances}$$

Assets are items that provide future cash flow or provide future economic benefits. Liabilities are claims on the assets. Equity is the difference between the assets and liabilities in for-profit organizations. Net assets or fund balances are the difference between the assets and liabilities in not-for-profit organizations.

To assess an organization's financial performance, a balance sheet is used. A balance sheet is a "snapshot" of an organization for a particular period of time (Dunham-Taylor & Pinczuk, 2010). It consists of assets, liabilities, and equity or fund balances. Assets include both current and long-term assets, investments, inventory, cash/cash equivalents, and accounts receivable as well as tangible assets (property and equipment) and intangible assets (no physical presence but do have value in the form of legal rights to use or sell). Liabilities also appear on a balance sheet and can be in the form of current liabilities (accounts payable, accrued salaries, other accrued expenses, government settlement accrual, long-term debt within 1 year) and long-term liabilities (long-term debt, professional liability risks, and deferred taxes) (Dunham-Taylor & Pinczuk, 2010).

Equity is another component of the balance sheet that includes either stockholder equity for for-profit organizations or fund balances for not-for-profit organizations. To gather the information about revenue sources, expenses, and costs of doing business during a period of time, a financial statement is used. It contains relevant information about the organization's ability to raise revenues, including provision of patient services and the coding of such services and provision of services for other healthcare facilities or investments. The financial statements will include costs and expenses, salaries and benefits, supplies, other operating expenses, and depreciation and amortization. Costs and expenses include such items as interest expense, equity in earnings of affiliates, settlements with the federal government, gains on sales of facilities, impairment of long-lived assets, restructuring of operations, and investigation-related costs (Dunham-Taylor & Pinczuk, 2010).

Another essential component of a healthcare organization's financial stability is its cash flow. The cash flow statements often include such items as cash accruals, bad debt expense, operating activities, financing activities, and investing activities. Additionally, all organizations must perform some type of internal accounting related to their cash flow, including their fixed versus variable costs, direct versus indirect costs, and activity-based costing and marginal costs. Fixed costs stay the same regardless of the level of activity (Dunham-Taylor & Pinczuk, 2010). Variable costs are those that change depending on the level of activity or volume (such as number of staff).

Creating the Budget and Knowing the Process

Most nurses are introduced to the budget process by learning about the organization's strategic plan. To successfully engage in the budget process it is best to work in partnership with members of the finance department, including the chief financial officer. Nurse leaders will have to develop the competency and capacity to share and support in the development of the staff's understanding of the budget and how it determines the allocation of resources for personnel, supplies, and medical equipment.

At the beginning of the budget process, projected costs of services are planned, submitted, and negotiated with executive administrators. Nurse leaders are often called upon to prepare an operating budget and a capital budget. An *operating budget* covers the day-to-day costs of a unit including such things as wages for regular and temporary workers, medical and office supplies, repair and maintenance, and the like. The *capital budget* covers the purchase of long-lived equipment (lasting at least 2 years) (Duhnam-Taylor & Pinczuk, 2010). It is developed separately from the operating budget and is often funded through separate sources, (e.g., capital campaigns, grants, etc.).

Most nurses will work with costs, not revenue; however, they need to know certain concepts such as revenues, which are charges made to patients or other clients, and accrual accounting records, which are revenue when it is earned (the service is provided), not when the cash is received. To effectively manage revenues, financial officers carefully price and package services that patients want to buy and insurance companies will pay for. Pricing may be accomplished in a variety ways: per patient per day, per event, or per unit of goods. Pricing must cover all costs, including direct labor, direct materials, and overhead. It is not based solely on costs, but on average, costs will define the lower bound of pricing (Dunhman-Taylor & Pinzuk, 2010). To *allocate* a cost (or revenue) it must be attributed to those costs (or revenue) billable elements of patient care. Nursing care is a billable service and requires budgetary information to formalize a department or cost center budget for personnel and other expenses beyond personnel including medical equipment and supplies.

Basic Unit-/Department-Based Budgeting

Today, nurses are expected to have some foundational knowledge in budget development and methodologies, including report formats, analysis rules, how to read a report, balance sheets, and cost report interpretation. In preparing a unit- or department-based budget, nurses must understand the operating expenses of nursing personnel, activities, and supplies. An operating budget has two main types of expenses: personnel expenses and nonpersonnel or nonsalary expenses. *Personnel expenses* (the largest part of the unit or department budget) include salaries and wages for hospital employees and contract staff, including overtime, shift differentials, holidays, orientation, education, in-service sessions, and benefits. *Nonpersonnel* or *nonsalary expenses* include medical supplies used for patient care (such as IV tubing and dressings), pharmacy costs for stock medications and syringes, office supplies, equipment rentals (such as copy machines), repair and maintenance of equipment used on the unit, and staff travel for educational purpose. Whether preparing a unit-based or departmental budget, nurses can review historical data to assist them in determining projected volume for both personnel and nonsalary expenses.

Table 10-4

Asking the Right Budget Questions at the Right Time
1. Do I have sufficient information about the needed nurse staffing to provide care for the patient population served?
2. How competent are the personnel assigned within the scope of my responsibility?
3. Are changes in the budget required to reduce costs and eliminate waste?
4. How would these cost changes impact the quality, safety, costs, and outcomes of care delivered?
5. What are fixed costs? What is included?

To prepare a nursing budget requires generating and controlling a review of past performance for either the unit, department, or division based on the nurse's position or scope of responsibility. The financial records from prior financial periods act as a basis for planning. The activities of the unit, department, or division will drive the plans for the projected financial period. The items in the major budgetary report that affect nursing often include hospital goals and projections. For example, a nursing unit was budgeted for 13 beds at 100 percent occupancy, but housed a census of up to 17 (130 percent) by using available swing beds. This census increased caregiver (RN, LPN, and CNA) hours per patient day.

The actual preparation of a new budget can be done based on a previous budgetary plan or a newly proposed plan (if a newly developed or modified service is considered). To complete the budget, a budget worksheet is essential. A budget worksheet is a a tool used by all managers to prepare their annual budgets. Most often than not it will include a number of columns such as (1) historic information from the old budget, (2) actual numbers with comments explaining the variances, and (3) revenues and costs. To be successful in the budget process, nurses need to learn to become inquisitive about the budget process and gain increased confidence in managing variances between the budget and actual costs, as well as asking for assistance by asking the right budget questions at the right time (see **Table 10-4**).

Cost–Benefit Analysis

Cost–benefit analysis (CBA) is an approach to evaluating and comparing the benefits and costs among two or more alternative programs or services (Penner, 2013). For nurses, cost–benefit analysis is a technique that may be helpful for determining the optimal size of a program or service or that may provide a framework for program evaluation or the financial analysis needed in a business plan. To fully appreciate the power of a cost–benefit analysis, nurses must convert resources and benefits into tangible measures that can be measured in dollars and cents. When considering cost–benefit analysis, nurses must identify the intended program outcomes or services, known as the *objective function*. The objective function must be measurable and demonstrate tangible gains in either reduced savings, increased quality, or increased patient satisfaction. An example of this may be the hiring of a lactation nurse to support a hospital's new designation as a Baby Friendly Hospital. The increased rate of breastfeeding mothers is an example of a measure of an objective function.

Costs are viewed as expenses or liabilities that produce the objective function of healthcare goods or services (Penner, 2013). These costs, related to goods or services, either may be measured in monetary units or can be converted into monetary units. Costs may be direct or indirect. Direct costs are those that are used in the production of an objective function. For example, the wages and benefits for the services provided by the lactation nurse are considered a direct cost. Indirect costs are those not used in the production of the objective function, such as the training and certification required by the lactation nurse.

When considering cost–benefit analysis, one must consider both the qualitative and quantitative benefits over time. Examining the net benefit of a given program, that is the total benefit less the total costs, provides leaders the ability to gauge the total impact of a proposed program. Separately, one can measure the impact of each dollar of costs versus the benefit it produces by dividing the total benefits by the total costs, resulting in an objective analysis of which allows for the comparison of different programs on an apples to apples basis. Ultimately in addition to quantitative measures, it is encouraged that leaders use qualitative common sense in judging the effectiveness of projects giving due consideration to the both the immediate and future results generated by a given program.

Using CBA allows nurses to gain the financial acumen and leadership to support evidence-based nursing practice while accurately measuring and reporting costs and benefits (Penner, 2013).

Financial Acumen and Leadership Capacity

Nurses, regardless of their position and title, must have the necessary financial acumen and leadership capacity to articulate business models for healthcare organizations. They must be able to interpret fundamental concepts of economics, understand general accounting principles, and define basic accounting terms. The financial acumen needed also includes the ability to analyze financial statements, manage financial resources by developing business plans, establish procedures to assure accurate charging mechanisms, and educate patient care team members about the financial implications of their patient care decisions. To effectively execute economically based decisions for patient-centered care that is safe, effective, timely, efficient, and equitable, nurses must understand their organization's mission and vision. This includes embracing the organization's core values, systems thinking, the need for collaboration with executive leadership, and effective teamwork. Each nurse must know how to build a business case for caring that is determined based on budget dollars available and how to best use those dollars to support and achieve the strategic plan. Financial decisions always occur within the context of the organization as a whole and often are tied to the organization's core value, such as "we will always do what is best for the patient." This value will drive every decision, including budget strategies.

All patient care services involve the economics of decision-making, whether that care occurs in medical-surgical units, critical care units, ambulatory nursing centers, diagnostic testing services, specialty clinics, primary preventative health clinics, schools, outpatient surgery, cosmetic services centers, outpatient dialysis units, or public health practice with the needs of vulnerable populations in mind. Thus, the economics of care is a part of the nurse's daily decision-making.

Nurses face the challenge of articulating what they do, how they do it, where they do it, with whom they do it, and the cost of that care. Specifically, nurses must be prepared to link healthcare outcomes to specific best practice nursing actions inclusive of cost. Nursing actions must be qualified and quantified, thereby rendering those actions tangible with specific attached value. Nurses no longer have the luxury of ignoring costs. To effectively manage costs and provide quality care services, nurses are expected to use barcoding and coding accuracy using ChargeMaster, examine and fix system problems, review how staff are utilized and scheduled, streamline and computerize documentation, and improve accuracy. By learning how to construct a business case for caring and creating a business plan, nurses demonstrate how they can improve quality and reduce cost (see **Table 10-5**).

Nurses with knowledge of informatics can relate nursing actions to cost and thus play an important role in bringing nursing to the proverbial economic "table." It is for these reasons that all nurses, as healthcare professionals, must be aware of the broader terrain of the macroeconomics of the time and how these broader issues affect and are affected by the microdecisions made in daily practice. Every nurse needs to be a nurse economist who will practice to promote efficient use of resources, both human and fiscal; standardize supply usage; and adopt a "just-in-time approach" to effectively lead change. The key

Table 10-5

Writing a Business Plan 101
A business plan should include the following components: • *Title:* Include the person's name who wrote the proposal with appropriate background information. • *Definition:* Define the proposed item, change, service, or program. • *Rationale:* Why is it needed? Why is this the best way? Outline other alternatives considered. • *Implementation plan:* Specify what needs to happen and the timeframe. • *Costs/benefits:* Show actual costs and how the proposal will change existing costs. Use a spreadsheet or table. • *Evaluation plan:* How will the effectiveness of this proposal be evaluated?

point to remember is that providing high-value nursing care requires the efficient use of resources. This means that nurses must learn how to identify and eliminate unnecessary waste, manage fluctuations in staffing, monitor budget variance, and reduce inefficiencies. Nothing else matters unless nurses appreciate the bottom line by ensuring quality while promoting safety and improving patient and staff satisfaction. The following case study is an example of this with a clear demonstration of the vital role nurse have in the economics and decision-making of the allocation of health care—decisions that include questions of access, quality, and costs.

Case Study

Impact of the Affordable Care Act by Linda Berger Spivack

The approval and anticipated implementation of the Patient Protection Affordable Care Act (ACA) has prompted states to face unprecedented budgetary changes related to structure and process. These improvements are expected to create new regulations in reimbursements to all providers of health care across the continuum. Individual states are also facing budgetary crises beyond the demands of health care that are driven by continued economic challenges. Responding to the fiscal shortfalls in their states, several governors are proposing budgets that significantly reduce reimbursements to providers including healthcare providers, specialists, hospitals, home care agencies, and rehabilitative and long-term-care facilities. Most states expect hospitals to see a drop in uncompensated care as healthcare reform through the ACA begins to become fully implemented.

In one state, the governor has proposed cutting approximately $500 million in hospital funding over the next 2 years. Each hospital must prepare for the impact and how these cuts will affect the unique operations of the individual facility. One strategy implemented in the state was the evolution of healthcare systems that have multiple hospitals, ambulatory care centers, home care, and long-term-care facilities. All members share in resources and all members coordinate care strategies and plans for expected savings, all while facilitating quality and safety measures. The bottom line is that the nurse leader must have a role in these decisions at all levels of administration from the bedside where the actual patient care occurs to the boardroom, where all the tactical and strategic plans for care begins.

Conclusion

The economic environment in which health care is delivered in the United States cannot be ignored. Nurses must understand the significance of the macro-level economic issues and how they influence the micro level of decision-making in clinical practice. Mannion, Small, and Thompson (2005) assert that the "power of economic ideas shapes the discourse of nursing and through this influences the choices and activities of nurses" (p. 370). Nurses can influence as well as be influenced by the realities of healthcare economics. Nurses must apply the macroeconomic view to the microeconomic setting in daily clinical decision-making. Nurse leaders must design and vigilantly monitor financial incentives to reward high-quality care, and organize the delivery system to ensure better care coordination that leads to a health system that produces the best outcomes for patients. This means creating structures that develop, nurture, and measure patient-centered care, including the need for daily collection of nurse-sensitive quality measures, such as pressure ulcers, falls, medication errors, and emergent care. Nurse-sensitive quality indicators can be used across the care continuum to help capture and demonstrate structural, process, and outcome measures that contribute to achieving patient-centered health outcomes. There is no time like the present and no better way to assume leadership for patient outcomes and advance health than for nurses to assume greater economic accountability.

For those nurses employed in healthcare systems like hospitals or home care, nurse-sensitive patient outcomes must become more visible and balanced with the economic interests and performance of the organization. Careful efforts must be made to address payment charges on healthcare organizations and create policies that will reward these organizations for investing in nursing and in the resources needed by nurses. This will become possible as more nurses lead change and advance health through innovations, improvements, and greater efficiencies, because inside every nurse is a nurse economist.

References

America's Health Insurance Plans (2013). *Age rating*. Retrieved from http://ahip.org/Issues/Age-Rating.aspx

Brill, S. (2013, March 4). Bitter pill: Why medical bills are killing us. *Time, 181*(8), 16–55.

Bush, H. (2012). Health care's costliest. *Hospitals and Health Networks*, 9(86), 30–36.

Centers for Disease Control and Prevention (CDC), National Center for Health Statistics (2003). *Personal health care expenditures of Medicare beneficiaries by source of payment, type of services, sex, race/ethnicity, residence and age, from the Medicare current beneficiary survey* 1992–2002. Retrieved from http://www.cdc.gov/209.217.72.34/aging/TableViewer/tableView.aspx

Centers for Disease Control and Prevention, National Center for Health Statistics (2006). State-specific prevalence of obesity among adults—United States, 2005. *Morbidity and Mortality Weekly Report*, 55(36), 985–988.

Centers for Medicare and Medicaid Services (CMS) (2010). *National health expenditure projections* 2010–2020. Retrieved from https://www.cms.gov/Research-Statistics-Data-and-Systems/Statistics-Trends-and-Reports/NationalHealthExpendData/downloads/proj2010.pdf

Congressional Budget Office (CBO) (2013). *The budget and economic outlook: Fiscal years* 2013–2023. Retrieved from http://www.cbo.gov/sites/default/files/cbofiles/attachments/43907-BudgetOutlook.pdf

Conover, C. J. (2004, October, 4). Health care regulation: A $169 billion hidden tax. *Policy Analysis*, 527. Retrieved from http://www.cato.org/pubs/pas/pa527.pdf

Conway, P. H., Goodrich, K., Macklin, S., Sasse, B., & Cohen, J. (2011). Patient-centered care categorization of U.S. health care expenditures. *Health Services Research*, 46(2):479–490.

DeBakey, M. (2006). The role of government in health care: A societal issue. *American Journal of Surgery*, 191, 145–157.

Dunham-Taylor, J., & Pinczuk, J. Z. (2010). *Financial management for nurse managers: Merging the heart with the dollar* (2nd ed.). Sudbury, MA: Jones & Bartlett Learning.

Emanuel, E. (2012, January 22). What we give up for health care. *The New York Times*, p. A4.

Ginsburg, P., Hughes, M., Adler, L., Burke, S., Hoagland, G.W., Jennings, C., et al. (2012). *What is driving U.S. health care spending? America's unsustainable health care cost growth*. Princeton, NJ: Robert Wood Johnson Foundation (RWJF), Bipartisan Policy Center. Retrieved from http://www.rwjf.org/en/research-publications/find-rwjf-research.html?at=Jennings+C

Graham Center (2005). Who will have health insurance in 2025? *American Family Physician*, 72(10), 1989. Retrieved from http://www.aafp.org/afp/2005/1115/p1989.html

Hartman, M., Martin, A. B., Benson, J., & Catlin, A. (2013). National health spending in 2011: Overall growth remains low, but some payers and services show signs of acceleration. *Health Affairs*, 32(1), 87–99. doi: 10.1377/hlthaff.2012.1206.

Henderson, M. C., Meyers, F. J., Ibrahim, T., & Tierney, L. M. (2005). Confronting the brutal facts in health care. *American Journal of Medicine*, 118(10), 1061–1063.

Henry J. Kaiser Family Foundation (n.d.). Health policy explained. Health care costs. Retrieved from http://www.kaiseredu.org/Issue-Modules/US-Health-Care-Costs/Background-Brief.aspx

Hogan, P., Dall, T., & Nikolov, P. (2003). Economic costs of diabetes in the U.S. in 2002. *Diabetes Care*, 26(3), 917–932.

Institute of Medicine (IOM) (2010). *The future of nursing: Leading change, advancing health*. Washington, DC: Author.

Lamb, E. J. (2004). Rationing of medical care: Rules of rescue, cost-effectiveness, and the Oregon Health Plan. *American Journal of Obstetrics and Gynecology*, 190(6), 1636–1641.

Mannion, R., Small, N., & Thompson, C. (2005). Alternative futures for health economics: Implications for nursing management. *Journal of Nursing Management*, 13(5), 377–386.

Moore, J., Salsberg, E., Wing, P., Dill, M., McGinnis, S., Stapf, C., & Rowell, M. (2005). *The impact of the aging population on the health workforce in the United States*. Albany, NY: University of Albany, Center for Health Workforce Studies, School of Public Health.

Nickitas, D. M. (2011a). Cost and coverage in turbulent times. *Nursing Economics*, 29(2), 57–58.

Nickitas, D. M. (2011b). Every nurse is a nurse economist. *Nursing Economics*, 29(5), 229, 250.

Nickitas, D. M. (2013). Health care spending: The cold, hard facts on cost, quality, and care. *Nursing Economics*, 31(1), 5–11.

Orszag, P. (2011). How health care can save or sink America: The case for reform and fiscal sustainability. *Foreign Affairs*, 90(4), 42–57.

Penner, S. (2013). *Economics and financial management for nurses and nurse leaders* (2nd ed.). New York: Springer Publishing Company.

Rice, E., & Betcher, D. (2010). Palliative care in an acute care hospital: From pilot to consultation service. *MEDSURG Nursing*, 19(2), 107–112.

Samuel, T. W., Raleigh, S. G., Hower, J. M., & Schwartz, R. W. (2003). The next stage in the health care economy: Aligning the interests of patients, providers, and third-party payers through consumer-driven health care plans. *American Journal of Surgery*, 186, 117–124.

Silver, N. (2013, January 16). What is driving growth in government spending? *The New York Times*. Retrieved from http://fivethirtyeight.blogs.nytimes.com/2013/01/16/what-is-driving-growth-in-government-spending/

Taylor, M. (2012). Hospital engagement networks: 10 big goals in 2 short years. *Hospital and Health Networks,* 86(5), 38–40,49–50.

U.S. Department of Health and Human Services (2013). *Read the law: The Affordable Care Act, section by section.* Retrieved from http://www.healthcare.gov/law/timeline/full.html

Weinstock, M. (2012). Who's in the driver's seat. *Hospital and Health Networks,* 86(5), 10.

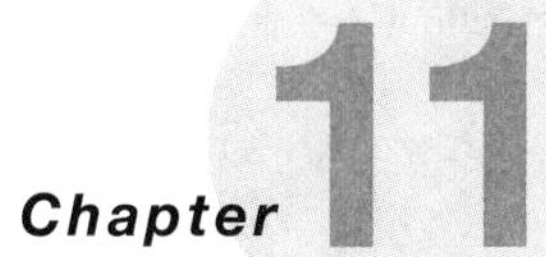

Chapter 11

Getting Involved: Public Policy and Influencing the Outcomes

Judith K. Leavitt and Andréa Sonenberg

What is public policy and why do nurses need to use the information in helping clients? At first glance, it seems like a curious connection, yet so much about the work of nursing involves decisions and influences beyond the nurse–patient relationship. Think about how many patients are denied or limited in their care because of lack of third-party payment from private or public insurance. What about the elderly client who is unable to get needed medication because the drug is not included on the formulary of their Medicare prescription drug plan? And what about the advanced practice registered nurse (APRN) who must give up caring for a particular patient because the APRN is not included as a preferred provider in the patient's health plan? These are real issues that APRNs must confront. The political strategies the nurse uses are the tools to support policy changes that enhance one's practice. One must ask whether the laws and regulations enable a nurse to practice to the full extent of her or his ability or if they place significant restrictions on practice. If the answer is that they are indeed barriers to practice, then the process of lifting such restrictions means that nurses and the profession must engage in political action to advocate for supportive regulatory health policy.

Certainly there is precedence for such involvement, as noted by Lewenson (2012). Our foremother, Florence Nightingale, was one of the first to argue for the need to change the larger sociopolitical environment to improve health, and Carper's classic 1978 work reinforced the concept of sociopolitical knowing as being crucial to practice.

Policy, Politics, and Values

Chaffee, Mason, and Leavitt (2012) use a framework to discuss the interaction of policy, politics, and values, which provides an understanding of how to incorporate knowledge about the policy and political arena in decision-making. *Policy* is defined as "principles that govern action directed towards given ends" and as a choice of action to achieve a particular goal (Titmus, 1974, p. 23). In public policy, it is the choices that the public and policy makers make about issues that affect the populace. Policy choices reflect the values of those who make the policies, the policy makers, who in turn are influenced by their constituents (Chaffee et al., 2012, p. 4). *Politics* involves the influences used to achieve the goal and always involve groups or individuals with different kinds of power; in other words, the groups with the most power and influence (be it resources, money, people, or connections) are going to be most successful in getting what they want.

All politics and policy take place within a particular value system. For instance, APRNs who advocate to prescribe medications as school nurses are assuming that parents and decision-makers support and value this aspect of the role. An example of the way that value system may be expressed is through supportive practice regulations that enable the APRN to independently prescribe medications for children enrolled in a nurse-managed school health center.

Another example is allowing APRNs to treat minors for a sexually transmitted disease. If the predominant values of state legislators oppose minors receiving care without parental permission, then APRNs will be unable to provide such care in that state. Unless nurses are aware of the predominant values of the public and policy makers around a particular issue, it may be fruitless to advocate a course of action, such as trying to get supportive legislation, when it is in opposition to prevailing values.

The Policy Process

To know how to resolve an issue, it is often vital to know whether there are laws and regulations that impede effective practice and if so, what they are. Therefore, to understand public policy, one must know how government works and how to exert political influence to get supportive policies.

How Government Works

There are three *branches* of government—executive, legislative, and judicial—and three *levels* of government: local, state, and federal. Health policy is made or determined by all three branches and at all three levels of government. For instance, practice issues are usually decided at the state level. State legislatures write and pass laws that define a nurse practice act for the various levels of nursing practice (legislative function), and state boards of medicine, nursing, midwifery, or education develop the specific regulations that give definition to the general outline of the law (regulatory function of the executive branch). For example, in New York State, the definition of the Nurse Practice Act in Article 139, section 6902 reads:

> The practice of the profession of nursing as a registered professional nurse is defined as diagnosing and treating human responses to actual or potential health problems through such services as case-finding, health teaching, health counseling, and provision of care supportive to or restorative of life and well-being, and executing medical regimens prescribed by a licensed physician, dentist or other licensed health care provider legally authorized under this title and in accordance with the commissioner's regulations. A nursing regimen shall be consistent with and shall not vary any existing medical regimen. (New York State Department of Education, 2011)

The law gives only the outline of nursing practice. The regulations spell out what is meant by case-finding, health teaching, and health counseling. The same section of the New York law defines nurse practitioner (NP) practice. Here is an excerpt:

> The practice of registered professional nursing by a nurse practitioner, certified . . . may include the diagnosis of illness and physical conditions and the performance of therapeutic and corrective measures within a specialty area of practice, in collaboration

> with a licensed physician qualified to collaborate in the specialty involved, provided such services are performed in accordance with a written practice agreement and written practice protocols. (New York State Department of Education, 2011)

Currently, amendment to this law is under consideration to remove the collaboration clause, which would expand the scope of practice of NPs to be consistent with their education and skill (New York State Senate, n.d., New York State Department of Education, 2011; Nurse Practitioner Association of New York State, 2012). A precedent has already been set in the state of New York by the passage of the Midwifery Modernization Act in 2010 (New York State Assembly, 2010), under which Certified Nurse-Midwives (CNMs) and Certified Midwives (CMs) practice independently and without the requirement of a written collaborative agreement with a physician.

It is the Board of Nursing (or in New York, the State Department of Education) that defines regulations like the "collaborative agreement." For instance, it would identify what the collaborative agreement must include, who can sign it, and how long it is effective. If the law states, as it does in New York, that an NP must take a pharmacology course to qualify for writing prescriptions, the regulations would define the kind of pharmacology course required to have prescriptive authority.

At the federal level, the Medicare law (Title XVIII of the Social Security Act) defines that an NP can be reimbursed for services; however, it is the Medicare regulations, which are promulgated by the Centers for Medicare and Medicaid Services (CMS) under the U.S. Department of Health and Human Services, that define exactly which services are covered. In the case of Medicaid, even though it is funded federally and includes some federal guidelines, it is managed by the states. Therefore, specific reimbursement policies under Medicaid are specific to each state. This contributes to the great variation in APRN practice and patient access to care across the 50 states.

Even the judicial branch of government influences health policy, primarily through enforcement of legislative and regulatory requirements. It is when these laws and regulations are challenged that the judicial system has the greatest impact. At the federal level, one of the most controversial decisions was *Roe v. Wade* in 1973. That decision, based on various amendments to the U.S. Constitution, upholds the right of a woman to make decisions about her own body. This interpretation thus conferred a woman's right to choose an abortion, if she so wished. Even though subsequent challenges have occurred with states placing more restrictions on abortions, the original decision still stands. More recently, the constitutionality of the Patient Protection and Affordable Care Act (ACA) was upheld by the U.S. Supreme Court (Supreme Court of the United States, 2011). Many stakeholders, including nursing organizations, supported Supreme Court consideration. This is an example of the role and power of the judicial branch in health policy reform and the influence of nurses, both individually and collectively.

The Federal Government

Washington, DC is the center of federal government where the legislative branch, Congress; the executive branch, the president and his or her cabinet; and the judicial branch, the Supreme Court, reside.

The Legislative Branch

The legislative branch consists of the two houses of Congress: the House of Representatives and the Senate. The House has 435 seats apportioned as a result of the U.S. Census, which is taken every 10 years. The number of seats in a particular state may vary depending on the number of residents in a state, but the total number in the House will always equal 435. House members are elected every 2 years, in November of an even numbered year.

The Senate has 100 members—two from each of the 50 states. Terms of office are 6 years. Approximately one third of its members are elected every 2 years. The political party with the majority of seats is known as the *majority* party for that calendar term (which is the 2-year term when members of the House of Representatives are elected).

The majority party elects a leader, who in turn appoints chairs of all the committees. This enables the majority party to have considerable political power in determining which legislation is introduced as well as which bills move through committees for a vote.

The primary role of the legislative branch is to make laws. Legislation is introduced by an elected member of Congress (at the federal level) and assigned to the committee in that house with jurisdiction over the issue. Legislators from each chamber often introduce the same bill simultaneously. Only a senator can introduce a bill in the Senate and only a member of the House can do the same in the House of Representatives. There are approximately 250 committees and subcommittees to examine the bills and hold hearings. In each session thousands of bills are introduced. Only a few make it through the complete process to implementation.

The majority leader in each house will determine which committees will have jurisdiction over the bill. Once a bill is introduced and sent to a committee, the chairperson will decide if and when hearings on the bill are held and what changes can be made before the bill is voted on by the originating committee. Often bills, such as those involved with health care, must be acted on by more than one committee. For instance, if a particular bill at the federal level concerned Medicare, it would be considered by the Energy and Commerce Committee as well as the Appropriations Committee. Although having different committees consider a bill can enable lobbying by more advocacy groups, it also slows the process toward passage or defeat. If a particular piece of legislation has money attached, it will have to be considered by the Appropriations Committee in each house. Members of the subcommittee on Health of the Appropriations Committee have a significant role in allocating revenue for each legislative proposal. For a fuller discussion of the appropriations and authorization process, see Hendrickson, Ceccarelli, and Cohen (2012, pp. 480–493).

The same bill must be approved by majority vote in both houses of Congress and signed by the president to become law. If a bill is voted down at the committee level or passed by only one house, the bill is considered "dead." Also, if it makes it through both houses of Congress but is vetoed by the president, it will not become law. The only way it could pass after a veto is if both houses override the president's veto with a two-thirds majority. Few laws are passed in this way, and usually only after the president has lost considerable power.

Executive Branch

The president, as the chief executive of the federal government, is responsible for overseeing the implementation and enforcement of federal laws. Through the cabinet officers and numerous agencies, commissions, and committees, the president creates regulations that define federal laws. For healthcare providers, one of the most significant is the U.S. Department of Health and Human Services (HHS) and its 11 operating divisions with over 300 programs (HHS, n.d.). These include everything from the Centers for Medicare and Medicaid Services to the Drug Enforcement Administration to the National Institutes of Health and the Public Health Service (HHS, n.d.). HHS provides funding for nursing education, as well as determines Medicare reimbursement policy. It also provides some federal mandates related to oversight of state Medicaid programs under the ACA.

Other important federal agencies involved in health care include the U.S. Department of Defense, which administers military health programs; the Veterans Administration; and the Departments of Education and Labor. Information about each is easily accessible online to determine federal standards, accountability, and program opportunities.

The power of the executive branch at the federal level emanates from the president's role in appointing cabinet secretaries with Senate approval. Because each serves under the direction of the president, department policies reflect the president's political and policy agendas. The other power of the president is in his or her ability to sign or veto legislation, particularly if his or her party has enough votes in Congress to sustain a veto.

Judicial Branch

The courts at the federal level have jurisdiction over matters that involve the U.S. Constitution and federal laws and regulations. The highest court is the U.S. Supreme Court, arbiter of last resort. There are 94 district courts where most federal cases originate. There are 11 federal appeals courts as well as two circuit courts. Although not traditionally thought to make policy, the judiciary branch has, in fact, been defining health policy through its decisions. For instance, the federal courts are increasingly becoming involved in labor disputes and medical liability issues, as well as issues of right to life and right to die (Keepnews & Betts, 2012). Legal scholars expect this trend to continue as states and the federal government create public policies related to privacy, liability, and public funding of health programs.

State Government

The structure of the state government is the same as that of the federal with several differences. All states except one, Nebraska, have two houses in the legislature, called bicameral legislatures. They may have a variety of names for their state legislatures, such as general assembly, legislative assembly, or the general court, but all are responsible for making state law, confirming governors' appointments, and approving state budgets. Most meet every year, though a few (including Montana) meet every other year. Some have a defined timeline, like a 3-month session (Mississippi), and others meet throughout the year, like California. State legislatures have jurisdiction over licensing and practice acts, most educational policies and funding, welfare and work programs, and numerous health programs, including public health and school health programs. Medicaid is a federal/state program, although states have increasing authority over the programs. The regulatory responsibility of the states is to develop rules around many of these issues, including nursing practice and the rights of patients.

Governors serve as the chief officer of states. More than half have lieutenant governors, the second in command, who may or may not be a member of the same political party as the governor. The power of the governor varies and is determined by the state constitution. However, as more decision-making has moved from the federal level to the state (devolution), governors and state legislatures have received increasing power to determine policy. All governors have the responsibility to propose a state budget and manage the budget after it is approved by their legislatures. They also have veto power over legislation. One of the most important political powers a governor has is to appoint heads of departments as well as governing boards who develop the regulations. One example is the board of nursing. In some states, certain department heads may be elected or appointed by one of these governing boards; thus the governor can influence the process through the appointment of the people he or she selects for governing boards. As a result, a governor can have considerable power over nursing practice.

Local Government

If it is true that all politics is local, the local government, because it is closest to the people, is the easiest to influence. The third level of government, the local level, has a variety of organizational structures and influence on health issues. Much is dependent on size. For instance, large U.S. cities, such as New York, Los Angeles, and Chicago, have city governments that are as complex as many states. A city government may administer its own Medicaid program as well as have considerable autonomy over public health. Most have jurisdiction over many aspects of public health, school policy, water and sanitation, and police and fire. Local governments administer school health through either local school boards or public health departments.

The structure of governance can vary greatly, from counties with elected boards like boards of supervisors to a single individual, the county executive or county manager. It is essential to know how your local government works to know how to influence health policies (Hendrickson et al., 2012, pp. 480–493).

Influencing the Process: Political Action

It is vital to know how government works and how public policy is made, but such knowledge has limited effect unless one knows how to influence the policy makers who make the laws and regulations that support patients and nursing practice. To have influence means to have power; to understand how to influence, one must determine who has power, what kind of power, and the extent of power in relation to others. Nurses and patients have power if they learn how to use it effectively. This is the essence of advocacy. (For more about power and political analysis, see Leavitt, Mason, and Whelan, 2012, pp. 65–76.)

Political Strategies

Political strategies provide the guidelines for decision-making and action. Strategies are most effective when carefully planned and done with groups of people. Rarely does an individual have enough power to influence a policy outcome. By working in coalitions with others who represent different constituencies, advocates can be more powerful in affecting policy. It takes persistence to keep policy makers focused on the issue. The most successful advocates are those who have a long-standing relationship with policy makers and can call upon them and keep them informed on a regular basis, not just at a time of crisis. For nurses, that means getting to know your legislators and representatives before you need them. Share your expertise about health issues. Invite them to your place of employment to understand the needs of your clients. When they get to know you, they will be more responsive when you ask for their help. Community Coalition Action Theory (Butterfoss & Kegler, 2009) posits that the success of a coalition is founded on the relationships among coalition members, as well as a connectedness with the community, learning and understanding the social context of the community, and establishing trust.

Legislation can take a long time to pass and be implemented. At the state level, it usually takes at least 3 years to pass. At the federal level, it can take much longer; for instance, the Family and Medical Leave legislation took 18 years. Policy reform to achieve equity of the Medicare reimbursement rate for certified nurse-midwives took 22 years (American College of Nurse-Midwives, 2010).

Persistence also requires that one offer solutions to issues, not just identify problems. Policy makers are rarely experts in health.

Consider these strategies for action:

- *Be prepared.* Be well informed on the issues, providing evidence on which to base any suggested reform (Clarke, 2012) and knowing the perspectives of different constituencies, especially the opposition. It enables you to prepare policy makers to respond to alternative arguments.
- *Frame the issue appropriately.* Place your issue in a larger context. For instance, if the issue is about insurance reimbursement, frame the issue as an "access to care" solution.
- *Work with others, preferably through coalitions.* Broad support for an issue assures a policy maker that they are taking the popular stand that reflects constituent support.
- *Know the goal—and be willing to compromise.* No legislation or regulation is ever agreed to without considerable changes.
- *Assess the timing for action.* Be sensitive to the larger political and policy environment to know when to push for an issue. If the values

of the public and the policy maker conflict with your issue, it might be best to move slowly in the beginning until there is congruence on the issue. However, always be prepared for a "full-court press" if it looks like there is support for the issue.

The bottom line is that the best health policy is only as good as the ability to get it implemented. Implementation requires a willingness to advocate for needed change, which is the driving force of political action.

Nursing Leadership in Decision-Making to Influence Policy Reform

This section offers the reader two case studies that highlight the decisions nurses can make to influence policy at both the local and state level.

Case Study 1

School Nurses: A Local Issue

Betsy Stand is a school nurse in a rural county of Mississippi. She covers four elementary schools with over 1,500 children. Because of the distance between schools, she spends one full day at each school and then divides the fifth day among the different schools. One of the policy issues that she confronts is medication administration. She knows as a registered nurse (RN) how important it is to know about each medication, each child receiving it, and the need to do an assessment both before and after administration. However, the school board has allowed secretaries and teachers to give the medications because the school nurse is not present when many of the medications must be given. Betsy had two events in the last month in which children had adverse reactions to the medications. One occurred because a wrong dose was given; the other because the medication had been discontinued, but the information was not given to the teacher who administered it.

Betsy needs to make a decision about how to handle the issue. How should she proceed?

Step 1: Assessing the problem: Betsy checks the medication policy and determines that it was developed by the school district; however, school nurse policy is developed by the Mississippi State Board of Nursing. She knows the Board is the regulatory agency for practice and any policy changes have to be approved by the full board. Members are appointed by the governor, usually with nominations from state nursing organizations.

Step 2: Information gathering: Betsy checks the Board of Nursing Web site for new regulations and then calls both the state nurses association and the state association of school nurses. She shares the problem and asks for their suggestions and help in devising a policy that is evidence-based (Clarke, 2012), safer for the child, realistic, and cost-effective. Both nursing groups agree to help find a solution for the problem.

Step 3: Developing a plan: Betsy asks for a meeting of nursing groups to develop a medication policy. Attendees included the executive director of the board of nursing, the president of the school nurse association, and the executive director of the state nurses association. They developed three different options for who could give medications: the teacher, a licensed practical nurse (LPN), or the RN. A grid was created to look at the costs, available personnel, and the chances of support and opposition for each. It was agreed that the most cost-effective, realistic option would be to recommend each school hire an LPN who would be required to take a prescribed medication course. She or he would be supervised by the RN who was responsible for that school. Although there would be an increase in cost for the school, the group was prepared to show that the cost would be offset by safety concerns for the students and decreased liability from potential medication errors.

Step 4: Gaining support: The three agency directors agreed to meet with the state Department of Education and the school board association about the issue. Betsy was to meet with the president of the local school board to apprise her of the potential policy change. Most agreed to the suggested change and were able to convince their colleagues to support the change. The executive director of the board of nursing then shared the information with the other board members. School nurses across the state were asked to send letters of support to state board of nursing members prior to their vote.

Step 5: Implementation: The vote was passed and the policy approved. Betsy and other members of the school nurses association worked on local implementation policies in each school district. LPNs were hired, and after 1 year there were no medication errors in any school district in the state.

Case Study 2

APRNs: Institutional Policy Supersedes State Regulation

This case study relates to an experience of several APRNs (the entire nurse-midwifery service) at a large teaching institution. Twenty-seven certified nurse-midwives (CNMs) were under the hospital department of nursing, five were clinical instructors in the department of obstetrics and gynecology (OB/GYN) in the university's medical school, and three CNMs were in private clinical practices. The private practice midwives had their own collaborating physicians and did their billing independently. They did, however, follow the same department-approved clinical practice guidelines as the two groups of service midwives. This included admitting and discharge privileges, attending births on the same labor and delivery unit, as well as conducting postpartum rounds on the inpatient unit. The only difference between them was their billing practice. Because the hospital CNMs were under the Department of Nursing, their general services were billed as a nursing component within the hospital room fee. This is not an uncommon billing practice for hospitals in charging for nursing care. As faculty of the medical school, the university CNMs had independent provider and Medicaid billing numbers, and had each of their attended births billed directly. For the hospital to be reimbursed for births attended by the hospital CNMs, as a separate service from the general "nursing care," their attended births were billed under the covering physician's Medicaid provider number. This is an illegal practice called incident to billing. It is illegal because the physician was not present for the birth; was often unaware of the patients' admissions, unless collaborating on a complication; and did not co-sign the note in the event of an uncomplicated labor and birth.

Someone in the hospital billing office reported the institution's billing practice to CMS, which subsequently charged the institution with billing fraud. A Federal Bureau of Investigation (FBI) investigation ensued. In response, and in order to be able to bill the deliveries under the physicians, the institution tried to revoke the delivery privileges of all the CNMs, not just the hospital group. Although the only difference among the groups was their billing practices, the institution claimed the reason for revoking CNM delivery privileges was because of adverse maternal and newborn quality outcomes as compared to physicians. The institution, however, would not provide any quality outcomes data on which it was basing the charge.

Because the private practice midwives had patients due to deliver, they immediately found other sites at which to attend births and did not participate in the ensuing advocacy efforts. The two hospital and university CNMs collaborated on advocacy strategies for their right to practice under their state licenses, as well as for their patients' right to access midwifery care.

Step 1: Assessing the problem: The first phase of the advocacy effort was to ensure patient care. The midwives, physicians, and nurses on the units reevaluated the flow of care on the labor and delivery and postpartum units, reassigning responsibilities for labor management and delivery to the hospital physicians. At a teaching hospital, there are several levels of providers who deliver care. In order to meet the patient care needs previously met by the CNMs, OB/GYN residents were brought from the main hospital and family practice residents, under their attending physician's supervision, were given expanded practice and unit responsibilities related to labor management and delivery. The university's graduate nurse-midwifery education program had to find other birth sites for students' clinical experiences. Simultaneously, the CNMs informed their patients that their births would be attended by physicians, which in many cases created a great deal of anxiety for the patients and their families, who had bonded with their midwives.

Step 2: Information gathering: The CNMs then met as a group and began to divide responsibilities to gather information about the claim of the physicians that resulted in their loss of clinical practice privileges. They needed evidence regarding: (1) CNM vs. medical doctor (MD) comparative birth data (vaginal vs. cesarean section; episiotomy and perineal trauma rates; complications of labor, delivery, newborn, and/or postpartum care), (2) state regulatory practice laws vs. institutional protocols, and (3) healthcare team response (MDs of various departments, RNs, educators) to the sudden change. In attempting to gather quality outcomes data, the CNMs approached the hospital and the university OB/GYN department. Both the hospital and the department refused to share the data on which they were basing the change in policies.

Step 3: Developing a plan: The CNMs continued to meet as a group, with six to eight of them taking the lead in organizing the advocacy efforts. The CNMs identified the stakeholders and developed a plan to seek their support, including the institution's other departments (pediatrics and school of public health), local and state legislators, national nursing and nurse-midwifery organizations, community advocacy groups, and the media. After agreeing on a timeline, the CNMs made a detailed plan and assigned responsibilities that included:

- Contacts with professional organizations
- Letter writing and appointments with local and state legislators and regulators
- Meetings with community groups
- Contacts with the media
- A process for keeping families informed and garnering their support

Step 4: Gaining Support: Once the CNMs identified the stakeholders, they delegated responsibilities to execute the plan, including:

(1) scheduling meetings with legislators (local and state); (2) meeting with the state Department of Education, through which the CNMs are licensed; (3) soliciting support from a variety of departments at the hospital and university, including the department of pediatrics, school of public health, and school of nursing; (4) contacting and meeting with national professional organizations, such as the American College of Nurse-Midwives and the American Nurses Association; (5) contacting pioneers and leaders in the fields of nursing, especially nurse-midwifery; (6) meeting with local community groups, especially those representing the majority of the patient base, which was Dominican; (7) soliciting the support of the media in order to publicize the occurrence, including print, radio, and television; and (8) informing their patients and families and soliciting their active involvement in the advocacy effort.

Step 5: Implementation: In meeting with the various stakeholders, the CNMs presented not only the published evidence of midwifery care in general, but also the evidence they had compiled from the hospital records that were available to them. They advocated for access to care for their patients, citing a history of documented outcomes and satisfaction from their patients. Some of the stakeholders (legislators, community groups, and the media) requested that the hospital and university provide evidence for the charges against the midwives. The institution was either unable or unwilling to provide the evidence. Several of the stakeholders, as well as the patients, put a great deal of pressure on the institution. Without its willingness to provide any evidence for rescinding the midwives' labor management and delivery privileges, the institution was hard pressed to keep the new policy. The midwives' privileges were returned to them, although with myriad restrictions. The limited privileges were in direct contradiction to the state midwifery scope of practice laws, as well as their credentialed skill based on education and board certification.

The advocacy effort took the midwives to local legislators' offices, the state capital; Washington, DC; the media; community advocacy groups; other departments in the institution; their patients; and their professional organizations. Ultimately, the CNMs won back delivery privileges, albeit with a narrower scope of practice. The collaborative group of 32 CNMs became a core group of about 6 to 8 doing most of the advocacy work.

The Licensure, Accreditation, Certification, and Education (LACE) Model (National Council of State Boards of Nursing [NCSBN], 2008) proposes to standardize education, licensure, and certification of the four groups of advanced practice nurses, of which certified nurse-midwives are one (NCSBN, 2008). The standardization of education and regulation of practice will, among other benefits, serve to unify the group in professional and patient advocacy efforts. Additionally, the Institute of Medicine report recommendations support the proposed standardization, while also recommending the reform of regulatory policies to allow APRNs to practice to the full extent of their education and skill (Institute of Medicine, 2010). Because the Affordable Care Act intends to optimize the role of APRNs as a means to expand access to primary care services, this case exemplifies the potential conflict of institutional policy superseding state scope of practice policy. It demonstrates how limits can be placed on APRNs and thus affect efforts to expand access to care.

These examples provide a framework for how nurses can use knowledge of public and institutional policy to affect change. In both situations, the nurses sought help and support from organizations and stakeholders that had an interest in the issue. They developed coalitions with these various groups, sought appropriate evidence to support their ideas, and made decisions accordingly that led to change. For the individual nurse, the most important decision was recognizing what needed to be changed to provide excellent health care and working with others and building coalitions and teams to expend the time and energy in advocating for the ability to practice to the full extent of their education and expertise.

Summary

This chapter focused on the ways in which public policy can inform nurses' decisions and how nurses can inform public policy. Nurses who are knowledgeable about the political process and who are active in the political arena use information about public policy to influence policy makers. The interconnectedness among policy, politics, and values was explored. The reader was presented with a short synopsis of how government works to form a basis for understanding how to affect public policy. Strategies for influencing policy makers were presented and two case studies provided examples of how nurses can use knowledge about policy and politics to support nursing practice and patient care.

Decision-making for leadership in nursing practice is a complex process that requires knowledge about many fields, which often includes health policy. Each nurse can find the tools to advocate for change, such as knowing how to work within multidisciplinary teams, how to use evidence to present to policy makers, how to work with the communities and families that may be affected by healthcare policy, and how to explore the legal, ethical, cultural, historical, and economic factors that impinge on the change sought. As we begin to incorporate this in our work, we will find that outcomes can not only improve patient care, but also expand our practice. It is empowering to know one has influenced legislation or regulation and even more so when seeing the benefits in improved health outcomes.

References

American College of Nurse-Midwives (2010). *Landmark health reform law to improve access to midwifery, benefit women's health*. Retrieved from http://www.midwife.org/acnm/files/ccLibraryFiles/Filename/000000000109/HR3590.pdf

Butterfoss, F. D., & Kegler, M. C. (2009). The community coalition action theory. In R. J. DiClemente, R. A. Crosby, & M. C. Kegler (Eds.), *Emerging theories in health promotion practice and research* (pp. 237–276). San Francisco, CA: Jossey-Bass.

Carper, B. (1978). Fundamental patterns of knowing in nursing. *Advances in Nursing Science*, 1, 13–23.

Chaffee, M. W., Mason, D. J., & Leavitt, J. K. (2012). A framework for action in policy and politics. In D. J. Mason, J. K. Leavitt, & M. W. Chaffee (Eds.), *Policy and politics in nursing and health care* (6th ed., pp. 1–11). St. Louis, MO: Saunders/Elsevier.

Clarke, S. P. (2012). Politics and evidence-based practice and policy. In D. J. Mason, J. K. Leavitt, & M. W. Chaffee (Eds.), *Policy and politics in nursing and health care* (6th ed., pp. 322–328). St. Louis, MO: Saunders/Elsevier.

Hendrickson, K. C., Ceccarelli, C., & Cohen, S. S. (2012). How government works and what you need to know to influence the process. In D. J. Mason, J. K. Leavitt, & M. W. Chaffee (Eds.), *Policy and politics in nursing and health care* (6th ed. pp. 480–493). St. Louis, MO: Saunders/Elsevier.

Institute of Medicine (2010). *Future of nursing: Leading change, advancing health*. Washington, DC: National Academies Press.

Keepnews, D. M., & Betts, V. T. (2012). Nursing and the courts. In D. J. Mason, J. K. Leavitt, & M. W. Chaffee (Eds.), *Policy and politics in nursing and health care* (6th ed., pp. 544–552). St. Louis, MO: Saunders/Elsevier.

Leavitt, J. K, Mason, D. J., & Whelan, E. (2012). Political analysis and strategies. In D. J. Mason, J. K. Leavitt, & M. W. Chaffee (Eds.), *Policy and politics in nursing and health care* (6th ed., pp. 65–76). St. Louis, MO: Saunders/Elsevier.

Lewenson, S. B. (2012). A historical perspective on policy, politics and nursing. In D. J. Mason, J. K. Leavitt, & M. W. Chaffee (Eds.), *Policy and politics in nursing and health care* (6th ed., pp. 12–18). St. Louis, MO: Saunders/Elsevier.

National Council of State Boards of Nursing (NCSBN) (2008). *Consensus model for APRN: Licensure, accreditation, certification, and education*. Retrieved from https://www.ncsbn.org/Consensus_Model_for_APRN_Regulation_July_2008.pdf

New York State Assembly (2010). *Midwife reform bill signed into law: Important step forward for women's health*. Retrieved from http://assembly.state.ny.us/comm/?sec=post&id=019&story=40267

New York State Department of Education (2011). *Education law: Article 139, nursing*. Retrieved from http://www.op.nysed.gov/prof/nurse/article139.htm

New York State Senate (n.d.). *S3289A-2011: Establishes the nurse practitioners modernization act*. Retrieved from http://open.nysenate.gov/legislation/bill/S3289A-2011

Nurse Practitioner Association of New York State (2012). *Legislative agenda*. Retrieved from http://thenpa.org/displaycommon.cfm?an=1&subarticlenbr=483

Supreme Court of the United States (2011). *National Federation of Independent Business, et al. v. Sebelius, Secretary of Health and Human Services, et al*. Retrieved from http://www.supremecourt.gov/opinions/11pdf/11-393c3a2.pdf

Titmus, R. M. (1974). *Social policy: An introduction*. New York: Pantheon Books.

U.S. Department of Health and Human Services (HHS) (n.d.). *About HHS*. Retrieved from http://www.hhs.gov/about/

Chapter 12

Use of Technology for Decision-Making

Christine Malmgreen,
Karen Koziol, Angela Northrop,
Veronica Elizabeth Francois,
Lorraine Von Eeden, Sharon Stahl Wexler,
and Lin Drury

Technology influences the way nurses make decisions, ultimately affecting quality and safety outcomes in health care. Information technology, in particular, supports the decision-making process. It supports the work of nurses at the point of service, in the classroom, in administration, and in research. To capture the essence and value technology brings to decision-making, the authors of this chapter provide examples of how technology is being used to improve health-care outcomes. Data mining, simulation, telehealth, electronic health records, electronic medical records, and virtual dogs illustrate some of the varied ways in which technology supports the education and practice of nurses. Several case studies in this chapter offer readers an opportunity to see the possibilities technology can bring to their decision-making. One final case study showcases the use of a virtual dog that has the potential to combat loneliness and isolation in the homebound older adult. Sharon Wexler and Lin Drury, two nurse researchers, lend a research proposal to this chapter that uses innovative technology that has the potential to support decision-making in nurses caring for older adults. Although their research is ongoing, the ideas they generate about the use of technology can help us think futuristically about integrating technology in nursing.

What Is Information Technology?

Information technology serves to facilitate decision-making in all practice settings. McBride, Delaney, and Tietze (2012) noted that technology has positive outcomes for nurses at the point of care. Simpson (2012) points out that value-based care initiatives emerging in the healthcare environment are rising in prominence for nurses. These initiatives provide an opportunity to lead a clinical practice revolution into a transformed environment of evidence-based, "better" practice decision-making. Technology, Simpson (2012) writes, "holds the key to making emerging better practices and the latest clinical breakthroughs available at the point of care" (p. 85). Simpson argues that technology can "push" the best evidence directly to the point of care, enabling consultation with the literature before making even the most complex clinical decisions. Value-based initiative efforts pair the United States' significant investment in health care with improved clinical outcomes. Simpson (2012) suggests that access to current literature at the point of care may serve to shorten the estimated 17-year lag between when clinical breakthroughs appear and when clinical practice finally catches up.

Nurses have the ability to provide care that is transformational with the aid of informatics. Cipriano (2012) asserts that nurses must implement strategies that enable them to access information, use evidence at the point of care, and ensure that they have the ability to *data mine* existing clinical data.

What Is Data Mining?

Data mining has many connotations. Anderson and Kotsiopulos (2002) define data mining as a "computerized technology that uses complicated algorithms to find relationships and trends in large data bases" (p. 2). It is digging into large data sets that, just like mining for gold, produces deep veins of data that can show patterns and generate knowledge to be used in practice (Wilson, Kelly, Lewenson, & Truglio-Londrigan, 2013). Data such as lab results, radiographic findings, demographic information, and invoice details are useful across all clinical specialties;

however, gaps remain in the awareness of data mining as a research tool and how to practically apply and integrate the knowledge discovered through data mining. Effective use of data mining in healthcare practice can support decision-making at the point of care by enabling the evolution of best practice, or practice-based evidence in combination with research evidence (Horn & Gassaway, 2007; Swisher, 2010). Nurses in hospital, nursing home, or community settings, already experts at recording their practice within medical records, can now be empowered to retrieve the data as trends of care and the impact on outcomes in a systematic, streamlined way that facilitates the speed, accuracy, and transparency of information flow.

Data mining can facilitate decision-making for problem solving in a structured way by identifying patterns that help gain a broader picture. Data mining promotes decision support because it can be predictive based on extraction and interpretation of information based on patterns. The decision support used to analyze raw data may be either fully computerized or a combination of human and computer activities. Clinical data mining allows for unanticipated findings because outcomes have already been entered. Epstein (2011) points out that using electronic health records (EHRs) for data mining has several advantages because of the nonintrusive and retrospective nature of looking at information entered during patient care as part of the electronic medical record (EMR).

The following case study demonstrates how mining electronic clinical records combined with easy access to electronic databases can improve decision-making at the point of care.

Case Study 1

Use of Data Mining Strategies by Angela Northrop

LS is a Bachelor of Science in Nursing (BSN)-prepared nurse certified in wound care. She was selected by her unit to become a clinical scholar on an evidence-based practice project and organized a team of two additional registered nurses (RNs) to assist her on this project. One RN was also wound certified and one worked as a charge nurse on an orthopedic unit.

In a team discussion they identified that they often saw deep tissue injuries (DTIs)—a first-stage pressure ulcer—in hip surgery patients during weekly skin rounds. As a clinical scholar, LS requested a nurse informaticist to data mine the EMRs to determine the prevalence of DTIs in orthopedic surgery patients during the previous 3 months. Examining EMRs within 24 hours post-op, the team learned that the incidence of DTIs among these patients was 18 percent.

Using the CINAHL (Cumulative Index to Nursing and Allied Health Literature) database provided by the hospital, the team did a literature search to determine best practices for prevention of pressure ulcers in post orthopedic surgery patients. They learned that putting at-risk patients on specialty mattresses immediately after surgery had the potential to decrease the incidence of DTIs.

The team prepared a protocol for the Post-Anesthesia Care Unit (PACU) nurses to screen for high-risk patients most likely to benefit from specialty mattresses. The proposal for the new protocol, and the data from the data-mined medical record, were given to the nurse manager, who used this evidence as a rationale to purchase these specialty mattresses for the unit. The screening tool protocol was entered into the EMR and would trigger an alert to the unit so that the unit nurses would get this information as soon as the patient was assigned to their unit.

To ensure compliance with the new protocol, the EMRs were again data mined and audited to ensure at-risk patients were identified and the mattresses were ordered appropriately. A monthly report from the Information Technology department that mined the records of all orthopedic patients revealed that within 3 months after implementation of the protocol and the alert and the purchase of the specialty mattresses, the incidence of DTIs dropped to 2 percent.

What Are Electronic Health Records and Electronic Medical Records?

According to the Office of the National Coordinator (ONC) for Health Information Technology, the EMR digitalizes patient records in physicians' offices and the information does not transfer outside of that office. In contrast, the EHR does that and more, focusing on broader health issues; it collects data that can be shared more easily among various stakeholders (Garrett & Seidman, 2011). EMRs were developed for the clinician's office to track clinical data over time and to monitor the patient's quality of care within the practice. The EHR goes beyond the capability of the EMR and provides the ability to share health information with other clinicians (Garrett & Seidman, 2011). They are both digitized records—an EMR is used in a single facility, like a doctor's office or clinic, and represents the digital version of the traditional paper medical record, whereas an EHR is digital health information (a record) that is shared among multiple agencies and facilities. Both the EMR and EHR are critical for the delivery of care that is seamless by bridging a practice gap that frequently involves communication. There are many examples of the delivery of this type of seamless care; however, an example that is evident in today's healthcare environment is the practice of medication delivery and medication reconciliation.

Various technologies may be applied and can help to bridge the communication gap among clinicians, thereby enhancing the delivery of care for complex medication processes such as medication reconciliation. This potentially can facilitate the prevention of medication errors, particularly in vulnerable populations such as community-dwelling older adults, and integrates the patient's health information across all disciplines of health care (Reich, 2012).

More specifically, in the United States, 90 percent of older adults take medications on a daily basis; nearly half (46 percent) take five or more. More than half of older adults (54 percent) have more than one doctor who prescribes medications, and about one third (35 percent) use more than one pharmacy (Stawicki & Gerlach, 2009). The Institute of Medicine (IOM, 2000) report, *To Err Is Human*, identified medication errors as the most common type of error in health care, resulting in as many as 98,000 people dying in hospitals within the United States each year. Medication errors due to multiple/chronic illnesses and normal aging changes put elderly patients at risk and can compromise their ability to engage in self-medication. Older adults use prescription medication more than any other age group; this increases the probability of adverse drug events (ADEs). An ADE is defined as any injury resulting from drug-related intervention/medication error or any preventable incident occurring during the medication use that may lead to patient harm (Pham et al., 2012). Polypharmacy creates a problem when elderly patients in the community are prescribed too many medications by multiple providers (Woodruff, 2010); this makes it very difficult to reconcile their medications and puts them at greater risk for ADEs. Technology may be used as a strategy to facilitate communication among providers, thus strengthening inter- and intrateam collaboration bonds to improve medication safety.

Technology such as that described can facilitate a healthcare system that provides seamless care without breaks and allows for better decisions to be made, thus improving patient safety.

The following case study demonstrates how potential medication errors can be prevented. It also illustrates how technology can facilitate better communication, and therefore better decision-making, among healthcare providers.

Case Study 2

Medical Errors Reconciliation by Veronica Elizabeth Francois

Electronic health records prevented an advanced practice registered nurse (APRN) from potentially placing an elderly patient at risk for a cardiac event. The patient was referred to the department for an adenosine stress test to get clearance for a hip replacement that was scheduled to take place the following week. An extensive medical history was taken, which included the names of the medications the patient was taking. At the completion of the medication history there was no indication that the patient could not undergo a pharmacologic stress test. Just before administering the test, the APRN check the Bronx RIO system (a secure system that allows clinicians of participating institutions in the Bronx to share patient health information) and found that 6 months ago the patient was prescribed dipyridamole by her general practitioner (GP). Dipyridamole, which is also call Persantine, can increase and prolong the vasodilative effect of adenosine and cause severe bradycardia and hypotension. When questioned, the patient stated she was, in fact, taking dipyridamole and the test was rescheduled. A near-miss like this example can be avoided if all clinicians use some form of health information technology to prescribe medications, access patients' health records, and share necessary patient health information to improve communication and collaboration.

What Is Telehealth?

Another important technology used in community healthcare settings to assist healthcare providers in their decision-making is telehealth. The Health Resources and Services Administration (HRSA) defines telehealth as "the use of electronic information and telecommunications technologies to support long-distance clinical health care, patient and professional health-related education, public health and health administration. Technologies include videoconferencing, the internet, store-and-forward imaging, streaming media, and terrestrial and wireless communications" (HRSA, n.d., para 1).

Telehealth (also called telemedicine) can be defined broadly as the use of telecommunications technology for medical diagnostic, monitoring, and therapeutic purposes when distance and/or time separates the patient and the healthcare provider (Hersh et al., 2006). This technology often is utilized to connect medically deprived or geographically distant areas with medical centers, to facilitate the provision of health services.

Telehealth enables healthcare providers to monitor physiologic measurements, test results, images, and sounds, usually collected in the patient's residence or a care facility. It is most commonly used for management of chronic diseases or specific conditions, such as heart disease, diabetes mellitus, and rehabilitation. Use of information and communications technology, such as cell phones, computers, networked devices, simple remote monitoring tools, and videoconferencing technologies, facilitates a "virtual visit" between the healthcare provider at the clinical site and the patient in his or her home.

The focus is on providing care in the home or community setting, with the primary purpose supporting the healthcare needs of the patient without disrupting his or her day-to-day life (Hersh et al., 2006). Physiological or symptom data communicated to a remote monitoring center can alert healthcare professionals when disease-specific clinical parameters are breached, thus affording the opportunity for earlier intervention, which might reduce the frequency with which expensive hospital-based care is required (Cartwright et al., 2013).

Telehealth facilitates a partnership between patients and healthcare providers. It plays a positive role in increased client self-management, including medication management and decision-making. Overall, the use of telehealth has advantages of not only improving clinical stability and addressing medication management, but also helping to improve clients' understanding of their medications, supporting client education regarding their health condition, facilitating client/caregiver support, and facilitating client safety in the home.

Case Study 3

Telehealth and Decision-Making by Lorraine Von Eeden

Consider the case of Mr. L, a 74-year-old man with a longstanding history of diabetes mellitus, chronic kidney disease, hyperlipidemia, and previous myocardial infarction with current left ventricular hypertrophy. Mr. L's daily medications include metformin, atorvastatin, furosemide, captopril, aspirin, atenolol, and losartan.

After Mr. L's recent hospitalization, the hospital's care management program enrolled him in its home-based technology program to monitor his clinical status for a period of 30 days post–hospital discharge (through use of audio/video monitoring). Vital signs and physiological measurements of heart rate, respiratory rate, blood pressure, weight, blood glucose level, and pulse oximetry were monitored on a daily basis by the program's registered nurse (RN). On the fourth day of monitoring, it was noted that over a 2-day period, Mr. L's body weight, heart rate, and respiratory rate were increasing, whereas his pulse oximeter values were decreasing significantly. Analysis of this online data by the primary health care provider and RN prompted the healthcare team to initiate a follow-up phone call in which Mr. L indicated that he was becoming short of breath and easily fatigued. Upon questioning by the nurse, it was revealed that Mr. L had only taken his medications for the first day post–hospital discharge, and had forgotten to take any medications thereafter. A diagnosis of congestive heart failure was made by the primary healthcare provider, who was able to immediately provide Mr. L with directions to increase the furosemide intake for 24 hours, and then to come into the clinic for a more in-depth medical assessment the following day.

Mr. L's vital signs were monitored via electronic telecommunication, with dialogue and interactive feedback provided through use of audio/video teleconferencing. The RN monitored the data and noted when the disease-specific clinical parameters were breached; she was then able to quickly initiate a follow-up interview to ascertain from Mr. L if additional functional changes were present. Based on feedback obtained, the RN collaborated with Mr. L and other members of the interprofessional team, and the healthcare provider was able to make a clinical assessment and develop a plan of care targeted toward resolution of these untoward clinical symptoms. Use of audio/video conferencing enabled the RN to guide Mr. L through the process of medication management, verifying exactly which medication he needed to take immediately and how many pills were to be taken, as well as to directly observe him taking the medicines. Mr. L was then given concrete instructions regarding a follow-up visit schedule at the clinic.

Mr. L's condition stabilized without need for hospital readmission. One week later, the RN and social worker conducted a face-to-face interview in Mr. L's home to ascertain his mental health status, as well as to determine if issues related to medication procurement contributed to his medication nonadherence. Issues related to Mr. L's medical insurance were identified; his Medicaid insurance was not active and Mr. L was trying to "stretch" the medicines out to last longer, thus resulting in missed and "forgotten" doses of medications. The social worker was able to initiate phone contacts with the Medicaid office to address the steps necessary to facilitate resolution of this situation. The RN reviewed all of Mr. L's medications, and re-emphasized the importance of him adhering strictly to the prescribed medication regime.

This case scenario illustrates the use of telehealth to facilitate early detection of a medication error (error of omission) via data analysis, and the prompt resolution of the ensuing clinical problem by enacting a concomitant change in medication dosage. Telehealth provided the infrastructure that facilitated implementation of the delivery of interprofessional team care, targeted toward resolution of untoward clinical parameters, with the goal of avoiding negative outcomes of early hospital readmission. The result of these actions was the prevention of more serious sequelae, including hospital readmission.

Use of Technology for Nursing Education

The emphasis on the use of information systems within healthcare organizations requires educators to become aware of the different technologies in use in health care today. Williamson, Fineout-Overholt,

Kent, and Hutchinson (2011) provided a rubric explicating innovative technology types with examples. They identified six innovative strategies with the potential to enhance quality and safe care by improving decision-making and access to knowledge, including simulation technology, mobile devices, social networking sites, the World Wide Web, clinical decision support systems, and EMRs. All of these emerging and evolving technologies have the potential to serve nursing and patient care by supporting workflow, enabling distant continuing education, facilitating interdisciplinary collaboration, and providing immediate access to resources for evidence-based practice (EBP) at the point of care.

One particularly significant development in computer technology discussed by Williamson and colleagues (2011) was simulation of the evidence-based decision-making process required in the clinical environment that can be developed in virtual and onsite classrooms. Simulation laboratories can be used by undergraduate and graduate students as well as nurses in clinical practice. This allows nurses who are seeking to improve their decision-making skills an opportunity to do so without the fear of inflicting harm. A case study follows that provides an example of this from an academic setting.

Case Study 4

Using Simulation to Improve the Decision-Making Skills of Nursing Students by Angela Northrop

Feedback from clinical instructors through an online survey at a college school of nursing indicated that some nursing students were slow to recognize an infiltrated intravenous line. The faculty and clinical skills lab faculty developed a simulation scenario with the following learning objectives. By the end of the simulation, students would be able to:

- Recognize when an IV is infiltrated.
- Perform the task of discontinuing an IV.
- Demonstrate therapeutic communication skills with the patient and other professionals in an interdisciplinary way.

The scenario contained specific assessment areas that involved varying levels of decision-making. During the handoff report, students learned that the patient was a 28-year-old female who was admitted 3 days prior. On admission she weighed 100 pounds. Two days prior to admission, the patient presented with cough, greenish nasal discharge, and low-grade fever. Her primary healthcare provider started her on oral antibiotics but the fever worsened. A chest x-ray confirmed pneumonia and the patient was admitted to hospital to start on a 10-day course of antibiotics. There was no history of asthma or any known allergies. She was currently being treated for streptococcus pneumonia with IV antibiotics and had an IV of normal saline running in her left hand. Hospital policy, based on best evidence, is that IVs are changed only if there is evidence of an infiltration and/or phlebitis. The student nurse must now assess the IV site on days one, two, and three.

Through the use of "time-lapse photography" embedded in the simulation program, the student nurse can see changes in the IV site and make decisions about whether to remove and replace the IV. In one scenario, the IV shows evidence of infiltration and the student must be able to assess this and then decide what to do.

High-fidelity simulation has turned a real clinical incident into learning scenarios. Video recording the interaction can be a powerful teaching tool. The simulations get more complex as the student's skill level grows. Using a simulated scenario operationalized through the use of computer technology helps the student learn how to make decisions at the point of care.

Researching Technology as an Intervention for Best Practice

In this final section we used the work of two nurse researchers who are studying the innovative use of technology to address isolation in older adults residing in their own home. These two researchers shared their proposal for a grant application that can lead to changes in the way decisions are made with regard to the care of older adults at home.

Case Study 5

"I Am Dougie, Your Virtual Service Dog": An Intervention to Address Loneliness in Older Adults by Sharon Stahl Wexler and Lin Drury

Overview of Research Program

This proposal will test an innovative intervention to reduce loneliness in older adults. Loneliness is a risk factor for ill health. Animal-assisted therapy is a proven intervention to treat loneliness, but not readily available to all who might benefit. A virtual service dog is now available on a tablet device to provide interaction 24 hours per day, 7 days per week. The virtual pet speaks in the language of the client, and responds directly to client questions and touch. The virtual pet displays a full range of emotions. A demonstration is available at www.gerijoy.com/video.

Loneliness is a demonstrated risk factor for functional decline and death in those over the age of 60 (Perissinotto, Stijacic Cenzer, & Covinsky, 2012). This is a problem for seniors living alone or in senior care facilities away from family and friends and while hospitalized. Families generally do not have time to visit every day, and with personal care attendants averaging $19 per hour, significant use of paid companionship is cost prohibitive for most Americans (Paying for Senior Care, 2012). Many seniors also resent interactions with paid caregivers. Even in senior care facilities, negative attitudes among the residents can stifle social interaction. Thus, to achieve the goal of healthy aging, new programs are needed to provide seniors with opportunities for social interaction and that are designed to improve mental well-being. Pet therapy has been demonstrated to be a cost-effective therapy that improves mood and is meaningful to hospitalized and community-based older adults (Kumasaka, Masu, Kataoka, & Numao, 2012; Coakley & Mahoney, 2009).

Description of Proposal

We propose to study an innovative method to provide companionship for seniors, in a way that is highly engaging and cost-effective compared to traditional means. The companions leverage the proven mental health benefits of pet therapy, taking the form of a virtual, dog-like pet displayed inside a wireless tablet device. In addition to life-like responses to multi-touch input, the pets are capable of intelligent, compassionate conversation. No typing or skills are needed to operate a tablet. Seniors speak to their virtual pet companion and the sound is transmitted over the Internet to specially trained staff. Thus, seniors are communicating with real people who are trained to effectively communicate with seniors and provide needed companionship. Because the virtual pet serves as an intermediary avatar, a pool of trained staff can be maximally utilized to converse with seniors on demand. On a broader scale, this could help to address the shortage of affordable senior care attendants and reduce the time burden for family caregivers. It will also reduce the strain on inpatient caregivers who are often thinly stretched and cannot respond as often as needed and implement psychosocial support.

A designated family member for each senior participant will upload family photos to the tablet. The virtual pet companion displays these photos to provide context for family-oriented, emotionally engaging conversations. For example, photos could be of the family pet, family vacations, or a recent marriage ceremony. Thus, 10 minutes of time by a family member can be leveraged into hours of family-based conversation in between visits.

Initial reactions from residents of nursing and assisted living facilities who have tried the virtual pet companion have been enthusiastic and positive. For example, nursing home residents have described it as "cute," "fantastic," and "priceless." The executive director of a five-star-rated skilled nursing facility noted, "After spending time with the virtual pet companion, the residents appear less agitated, more engaged in conversation, and in a happier emotional state."

During this study, we will compare six older adult patients representing two distinct populations: homebound older adults and hospitalized older adults. We will address four health outcomes: (1) sense of social isolation, (2) depression, (3) mental well-being, and (4) cognitive functioning. Instruments validated in older populations will be administered before, during, and after the intervention to assess potential changes in each outcome. Standard geriatric scales such as the Geriatric Depression Scale (GDS) and Mini Mental State Exam (MMSE) will be used to determine potential improvements in depression and cognitive function. The Pleasure-Arousal-Dominance (PAD) and Positive and Negative Affect Schedule (PANAS) will be used to determine how participants' emotional health changes over the course of the study.

We will use a randomized controlled trial design that randomly assigns participants to either a control group (no virtual pet companion) or an intervention group (uses virtual pet companion). All participants will be asked to complete the assessments before, during, and after the study period. Seniors will participate in the program for 3 months. We will compare results between the two populations for both experimental and control groups.

Conclusion

The case studies presented here demonstrate how decision-making skills for educators, nurse researchers, nursing students, and nurses in clinical practice can be amplified by technology. Educators can use simulation to create scenarios that enable students to practice decision-making about clinical care. Nurses in practice, in academia, and in research settings have access to electronic databases and the ability to data mine to build evidence-based practice. Data mining, electronic databases, simulation technology, EHR, EMR, and computers are just some examples of technology that contemporary nurses have at their disposal to enhance decision-making and improve care. Just as there is a range of practice settings and processes of decision-making, there is a range of technology, information literacy, and methodologies available. Innovative use of technology in caring for individuals, families, communities, and populations is necessary, and nurses need to be innovative in the way they approach and use technology.

References

Anderson, J., & Kotsiopulos, A. (2002). Enhanced decision making using data mining: Applications for retailers. *Journal of Textile and Apparel Technology and Management*, 2(3), 1–14.

Cartwright, M., Hirani, S. P., Rixon, L., Beynon, M., Doll, H., Bower, P., et al. (2013). Effect of telehealth on quality of life and psychological outcomes over 12 months (Whole Systems Demonstrator telehealth questionnaire study): Nested study of patient reported outcomes in a pragmatic, cluster randomized controlled trial. *British Medical Journal*, 346, 1–20.

Cipriano, P. (2012). The importance of knowledge-based technology. *Nursing Administration Quarterly*, 36(2), 136–146.

Coakley, A. B., & Mahoney, E. K. (2009). Creating a therapeutic and healing environment with a pet therapy program. *Complementary Therapies in Practice*, 15, 141–146. doi: 10.1016/j.ctcp.2009.05.004.

Epstein, I. (2011). Reconciling evidence-based practice, evidence-informed practice, and practice-based research: The role of clinical data-mining. *Social Work*, 56(3), 284–288.

Garrett, P., & Seidman, J. (2011, January 4). *EMR vs EHR—What is the difference?* Health IT Buzz. Washington, DC: U.S. Department of Health and Human Services. Retrieved from http://www.healthit.gov/buzz-blog/electronic-health-and-medical-records/emr-vs-ehr-difference/

Health Resources and Services Administration (HRSA), Rural Health (n.d.). *Telehealth*. Retrieved from http://www.hrsa.gov/ruralhealth/about/telehealth/

Hersh, W. R., Hickam, D. H., Severance, S. M., Dana, T. L., Krages, K. P., & Helfand, M. (2006). *Telemedicine for the Medicare population: Update*. Evidence Reports/Technology Assessments, No. 131. Rockville, MD: Agency for Healthcare Research and Quality.

Horn, S., & Gassaway, J. (2007). Practice-based evidence study design for comparative effectiveness research. *Medical Care*, 45(10), S50–S57. doi: 10.1097/MLR.0b013e318070c07b.

Institute of Medicine (IOM) (2000). *To err is human: Building a safer health system*. Washington, DC: National Academies Press.

Kumasaka, T., Masu, H., Kataoka, M., & Numao, A. (2012). Changes in patient mood through animal-assisted activities in a palliative care unit. *International Medical Journal*, 19(4), 333–337.

McBride, S., Delaney, J., & Tietze, M. (2012). Health information technology and nursing. *American Journal of Nursing*, 112(8), 36–44.

Paying for Senior Care (2012). *Financial options to help pay for or reduce the cost of home care*. Retrieved from http://www.payingforseniorcare.com/longtermcare/paying-for-home-care.html

Perissinotto, C. M., Stijacic Cenzer, I., & Covinsky, K. E. (2012). Loneliness in older persons: A predictor of functional decline and death. *Archives of Internal Medicine*, 172(14), 1078–1083.

Pham, J. C., Aswani, M. S., Rosen, M., Lee, H., Huddle, M., Weeks, K., et al. (2012). Reducing medical errors and adverse events. *Annual Review of Medicine*, 63, 447–463. doi: 10.1146/annurev-med-061410-121352.x.

Reich, A. (2012). Discipline doctors: The electronic medical record and physicians' changing relationship to medical knowledge. *Social Science and Medicine*, 74, 1021–1028. doi: 10.1016/j.socscimed.2011.12.032.

Simpson, R. L. (2012). Technology enables value-based nursing care. *Nursing Administration Quarterly*, 36(1), 85–87.

Stawicki, S. P., & Gerlach, A. T. (2009). Polypharmacy and medication errors: Stop, listen, look, and analyze. *OPUS12 Scientist*, 3, 6–10.

Swisher, A. K. (2010). Practice-based evidence [editorial]. *Cardiopulmonary Physical Therapy Journal*, 21(2), 4.

Williamson, K. M., Fineout-Overholt, E., Kent, B., & Hutchinson, A. M. (2011, fourth quarter). Teaching EBP: Integrating technology into academic curricula to facilitate evidence-based decision-making. *Worldviews on Evidence-Based Nursing*, 8(4), 247–251.

Wilson, M. L., Kelly, M., Lewenson, S. B., & Truglio-Londrigan, M. (2013). Informatics in public health nursing. In M. Truglio-Londrigan, & S. B. Lewenson (Eds.), *Public health nursing: Practicing population-based care* (2nd ed., pp. 151–177). Burlington, MA: Jones & Bartlett Learning.

Woodruff, K. (2010). Preventing polypharmacy in older adults. *American Nurse Today*, 5(10). Retrieved from http://www.americannursetoday.com/article.aspx?id=7132&fid=6852#

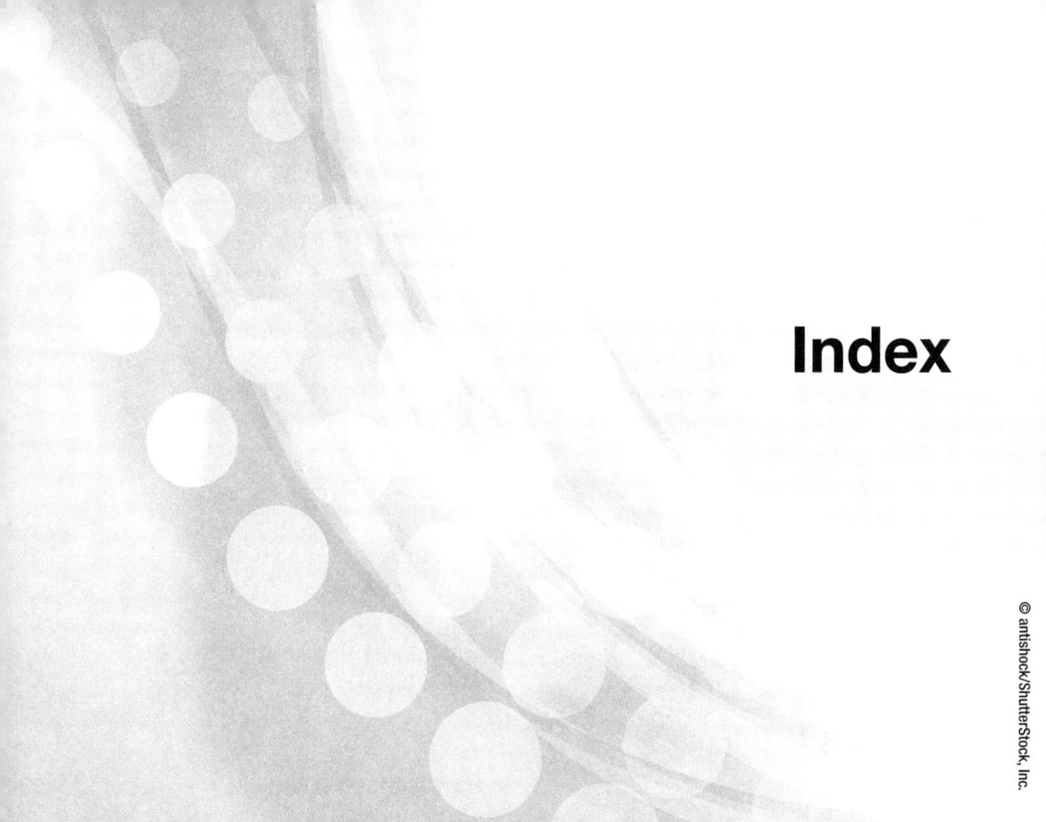

Index

Note: Page numbers followed by f and t indicate material in figures and tables respectively.

A

B

I

N

S